Keto Diet
Book FOR BEGINNERS UK

Eating Keto is simple Less carbs, more healthy fats, Easy and delicious
320 recipes Incl. 5 Week Special Meal Plan

ISBN: 9798832651958

TABLE OF CONTENTS

Introduction

Despite continuous advances in the medical world, obesity remains a significant worldwide health hazard, with adult mortality of 2.8 million per year. The majority of chronic diseases like diabetes, hypertension, and heart disease are primarily related to obesity which is usually a product of an unhealthy lifestyle and poor dietary habits. Appropriately tailored diet regimens for weight reduction can help manage the obesity epidemic to some extent. One diet regimen that has proven to be very effective for rapid weight loss is a very-low-carbohydrate and high-fat ketogenic diet

What is keto?

The Keto, or ketogenic, diet is a diet that significantly restricts the number of carbohydrates consumed while promoting moderate eating amounts of protein and higher amounts of fat.

Originally the diet was developed as a treatment for Epilepsy in young children as an alternative to the popular treatment of simply fasting. This is because the altered sugar/fat levels affect the excitability of the brain, which can, in turn, have a positive impact on the frequency/severity of seizures.

The ketogenic diet consists of 6% carbohydrates, 60% fats, and 34% protein. As the diet is deficient in carbohydrates, the body cannot use glucose (which comes from carbs) as an energy source, and it is forced to find an alternative energy source. As a result, the liver produces some substances called ketone bodies that are used as the new energy source. At this stage, the body enters a state called ketosis and becomes much more effective at burning fats. Any other ketone bodies not used as an energy source are removed via urine and sweat.

Types of keto diets

There are several categories of the ketogenic diet, some of which are:

The standard ketogenic diet obtains about 75 percent of your calories from fat (i.e., oils, fatty meat or fish, etc.), 20 percent from protein, and 5 percent from carbohydrates.

A cyclical ketogenic diet allows some days of higher carb intake. For instance, if you find it hard to stick to a very low-carb diet every day, you can practice five ketogenic days followed by two high-carb days. This is an appropriate approach when you start keto and your body is still adjusting to the diet.

A targeted ketogenic diet offers you to increase carb consumption around workouts.

A high protein ketogenic diet includes a higher protein intake with a ratio of 60% fat, 35% protein, and 5% carbs.

Benefits of a keto diet

Summer barbeques are coming to an end, and the holiday season is just around the corner. Are you worried about losing a few extra pounds for the Christmas card photo? Or maybe you over-did at the cookouts already, and now you want to drop a little weight before you need stretch pants by the New Year. Keto has become a trendy diet choice for rapid weight loss. With popular diets like Adkins, and celebrity endorsements, like Melissa McCarthy, it can be exciting to think of what this diet can do for you. Influential groups, like Love Yourself, provide Keto meals pre-portioned and delivered to your home. Perfect for losing weight without all the extra prep. There are some skeptics about the health benefits of Keto, but there is evidence to support several additional benefits of following a ketosis diet.

Rapid Weight Loss

Of course, the first benefit of following a Keto diet is rapid weight loss. Of all recommended diets, Keto provides the most dramatic weight loss. One study found that Keto had the most weight loss over the first 4-6 months vs. a low-fat diet and even the Mediterranean Diet, often prescribed for patients with high blood pressure or cardiac issues. Long-term dieting with Keto even provides more weight loss after two years.

It helps your cholesterol

In a medical study in 2004, the benefits of Keto were studied over 24 weeks. They found that in the first eight weeks of the Keto diet, there was a significant decrease in LDL and total cholesterol in the patients in the study. HDL, the good cholesterol, improved week over week for the 24-week study. So even though the diet is high in fat, which can be concerning to someone with high cholesterol, there is evidence that this diet could help improve your numbers in the short term. (et.al, 2004)

Reduced Triglycerides

Triglycerides are a type of lipid (fat) found in your blood, and having a high triglyceride level in your blood can increase your heart disease and stroke risk. In the same study of patients on the keto diet, it was observed that triglyceride levels also decreased week after week for the entire 24-week study.

Suppresses hunger

Ketones influence the hormones which control your appetite. Ketones increase cholecystokinin (CCK) and suppress ghrelin (hunger hormones), which lets your brain know when you have eaten enough. The result of this is rapid weight loss.

Reduces inflammation

The keto diet is an anti-inflammatory and can protect you against major degenerative diseases such as cancer and Alzheimer's.

Increases energy

Ketosis enables the brain to create more power generators within your cells, allowing you to have more energy to use during the day.

Blood glucose control

One of the best benefits of a keto diet is that since it is low-carb, it is a very diabetic-friendly diet. Patients who have been on this diet have lost weight, decreased their blood glucose, and sometimes have even been able to come off their medications. Low carb diets, like keto, are highly recommended for those with diabetes. If you are pre-diabetic, it is the best time to start a keto diet; it could help you avoid ever needing to use insulin to control your blood sugar.

What is ketosis? And how do you know if you're in it?

If you follow the recommended foods to eat and avoid as stated above, then your body should enter ketosis. That's the metabolic state where your body uses fat for fuel instead of carbohydrates. To ensure that the diet you're following has the right effect on your body, you can check you are in ketosis with testing kits, such as urine strips, breath analyzers, and blood tests, which you can purchase online.

These tests can give you an accurate reading. However, there are some signs of being in ketosis that you can use as a guideline:

- Increased urination can occur in the early stages
- Increased thirst
- A fruity taste in the mouth/bad breath
- Decreased hunger or appetite

What Foods to eat

Fats, proteins, and minimal carbs are what you need to eat to be successful on keto. Carbs will make up a significantly smaller portion of your diet on keto than on an average eating plan.

Here is a breakdown of some of the foods you'd eat on keto:

Fats: 70-80%	Protein: 10-20%	Carbs: 5-10%
Butter	Beef	Leafy green vegetables
Bacon	Poultry	(these are the most keto-
Avocado	Pork	approved veggies)
Oils – coconut, olive, etc.	Lamb	Broccoli
Ghee	Organ meats	Asparagus
Cheese	High-fat dairy	Mushrooms
Animal fats – duck fat,	Eggs	Herbs

lard, etc.	Deli meat	Berries and other low-sugar fruits
Pork rinds	Fatty fish	
Nuts	Seafood	
Seeds		

For a typical 2,000 calorie per day diet, this translates to about:

- 165 grams of fat
- 75 grams of protein
- 20-30 grams of carbs

What Foods to avoid

For keto to work correctly, a dramatic decrease in carbs is required. Carbs can be found in a wide variety of foods that you would need to eliminate from your diet, including:

- Grains, such as bread, pasta, and rice
- High-sugar fruits including oranges, apples, grapes, pears, bananas, and mangos
- Vegetables with a high starch content, such as potatoes, sweet potatoes, and parsnips
- Legumes including beans, chickpeas, and lentils
- Sugary drinks such as fizzy drinks, fruit juices, energy drinks, and alcohol

Some are concerned that cutting some of these foods means missing out on the broader nutrient benefit of these foods.

Take, for example, the salad below. It looks healthy, right? It's got tonnes of broccoli, as well as mushrooms and seeds. It's also called 35.5g of carbs per serving, which would exceed the amount you are allowed to eat on keto.

Why should I consider going keto?

Getting started on a keto diet plan can have many benefits depending on your specific goals. It is undertaken by many as a method for weight loss and has shown some very successful results! It appears that weight can be lost at a more rapid level when undertaking a keto diet over most others (for example, a low-fat diet) due to fat stores being used to burn energy.

When shifting from a typically 'unhealthy' diet in the hopes of losing weight, many individuals 'fall off the wagon' after restricting themselves from consuming their favourite foods and swapping incredibly filling, high-fat foods such as burgers, bacon, and pizzas for low-calorie salads and lean meats. This is where keto can step in to help! Where most diets restrict fats, keto promotes their consumption! That means that indulgent ingredients like steak, cream, and cheese are promoted as components within the diet and can be consumed without any restriction!

Keto flu

There is also anecdotal evidence to suggest a keto diet could cause many other side effects - collectively referred to as 'keto flu'; however, these seem to end within a few weeks.

Possible side effects can include:

- Headaches
- Fatigue
- Nausea
- Dizziness
- "Brain fog"
- Gastrointestinal discomfort
- Decreased energy
- Feeling faint
- Sleep issues
- Diarrhea, constipation, and vomiting

While on the keto diet, monitor any symptoms like these and ensure you're staying hydrated. You could ease into a ketogenic diet by following a low-carb diet for a few weeks and then switch over to full keto

Keto tips and tricks

Although getting started on the ketogenic diet can be challenging, there are several tips and tricks that you can use to make it easier.

- Start by familiarizing yourself with food labels and checking the grams of fat, carbs, and fiber to determine how your favorite foods can fit into your diet.
- Planning out your meals in advance may also help you save extra time throughout the week.
- Many websites, food blogs, apps, and cookbooks also offer keto-friendly recipes and meal ideas that you can use to build your custom menu.
- Alternatively, some meal delivery services even offer keto-friendly options for a quick and convenient way to enjoy keto meals at home.
- Look into healthy frozen keto meals when you're short on time
- When going to social gatherings or visiting family and friends, you may also want to consider bringing your food, making it easier to curb cravings and stick to your meal plan.

Frequently asked questions

Here are answers to some of the most common questions about the ketogenic diet.

Can I ever eat carbs again?

Yes. However, it's essential to reduce your carb intake initially significantly. After the first 2 to 3 months, you can eat carbs on special occasions and return to the diet immediately afterward.

Will I lose muscle?

There's a risk of losing some muscle on any diet. However, protein intake and high ketone levels may help minimize muscle loss, especially if you lift weights.

How much protein can I eat?

Protein should be moderate, as a very high intake can spike insulin levels and lower ketones. Around 35% of total calorie intake is probably the upper limit.

What if I am constantly tired, weak, or exhausted?

You may not be in full ketosis or be utilizing fats and ketones efficiently. To counter this, lower your carb intake and revisit the points above. A supplement like MCT oil or ketones may also help.

My urine smells fruity. Why is this?

Don't be alarmed. This is simply due to the excretion of by-products created during ketosis.

My breath smells. What can I do?

This is a common side effect. Try drinking naturally flavored water or chewing sugar-free gum.

I heard ketosis was extremely dangerous. Is this true?

People often confuse ketosis with ketoacidosis. Ketoacidosis is dangerous, but ketosis on a ketogenic diet is usually fine for healthy people. Speak to your doctor before starting any new diet.

I have digestion issues and diarrhea. What can I do?

This common side effect usually passes after 3 to 4 weeks. If it persists, try eating more high fiber veggies

The 35-day meal plan

Now, the moment you've been waiting for – the meal plan! This chapter will find a 35-day meal plan for the standard ketogenic diet, divided into four weeks. Every day, you'll follow the procedure to eat breakfast, lunch, dinner, and a snack or dessert with a calorie range between 1,800 and 2,000.

One thing I want to mention before you get started is net carbs.

Many people who follow the ketogenic diet prefer to track net carbs rather than total carbs. To calculate net carbs, you simply take the total carb count of the meal and subtract the grams of fiber since fiber cannot be digested. I prefer to track total carbs like what I have mentioned in my first book, but I have included the grams of fiber and net carbs in these recipes, so you can choose which way to go.

I prefer more buffer for the carb count because I want to reduce the number of obstacles keeping me from ketosis. Many of my readers and friends have raised this point, and you can be sure quite a few nights or afternoons were spent in heated debate! Okay, it wasn't that serious, but it sufficed to say that many discussions went into this topic. Therefore, I thought it might be better if I gave you a say in this net carb-total carb debate. You get to choose whichever you prefer. In my personal opinion, when you are in the initial stages of trying to enter ketosis, keeping your total carb count in mind is probably one of the better practices you can adopt. A 20 to 50-gram range of carbs would usually work to push the body into a ketogenic state.

After you have gotten keto-adapted and the body gets used to burning fat for fuel, you can then start to bring net carbs into the equation.
Keep in mind the calorie range for these meal plans – if you read my first book and calculate your own daily caloric needs, you may need to make some adjustments. If you're trying the ketogenic diet for the first time, however, it may be easiest to follow the plan as is until you get the hang of it.
The first week of this 28-day meal plan is designed to be incredibly simple in meal prep to focus on learning which foods to eat and which to avoid on the ketogenic diet – that's why you'll find more smoothies and soups here than in the following weeks. If you finish the first week and feel like you still need some time to adjust keto, feel free to repeat it before moving on to week two. The meal plans also consider leftovers and the yields of various recipes to have minimal waste from your efforts in the kitchen. So, without further ado, let's take a look at the meal plans

35-Days Keto Diet Weight Loss Challenge

First Week Meal Plan

DAYS	BREAKFAST	LUNCH	DINNER
Sunday	Keto meatloaf muffins Page NO- 21	Keto pork chops with asparagus Page NO- 54	Seafood salad with Avocado Page NO- 64
Monday	Loaded keto breakfast wrap Page NO-22	Keto Caesar salad Page NO- 41	Keto oven-baked Brie cheese Page NO- 64
Tuesday	Keto egg muffins Page NO- 34	Keto fried salmon with Asparagus Page NO- 40	1/2 amount of Low-carb pumpkin soup Page NO- 68
Wednesday	Butter "bulletproof" coffee Page NO- 30	Keto tuna salad with poached eggs Page NO- 57	Keto Thai fish curry and bok choy Page NO- 55
Thursday	Classic bacon and eggs Page NO- 25	Yogurt chicken kebabs with beet carpaccio Page NO- 46	Keto oven-baked Brie Cheese Page NO- 64
Friday	Keto meatloaf muffins Page NO- 21	Shrimp salad with hot bacon fat dressing Page NO- 59	1/2 amount of Keto pizza Page NO- 65
Saturday	Butter "bulletproof" coffee Page NO- 30	Keto Tex-Mex burger Plate Page NO- 50	Creamy low-carb broccoli Page NO- 69

35-Days Keto Diet Weight Loss Challenge

Second Week Meal Plan

DAYS	BREAKFAST	LUNCH	DINNER
Sunday	Keto breakfast tapas Page NO-22	Keto Italian cabbage stir-fry Page NO- 63	Keto deviled eggs Page NO- 70
Monday	Butter "bulletproof" coffee Page NO-30	Keto pork chops with blue-cheese sauce Page NO- 49	Keto baked salmon with Pesto and broccoli Page NO- 70
Tuesday	Keto breakfast tapas Page NO-22	Keto ground beef and broccoli Page NO-49	Salad Niçoise Page NO- 56
Wednesday	Keto meatloaf muffins Page NO-21	Keto Caesar salad Page NO- 41	Keto tuna plate Page NO- 68
Thursday	Salad sandwiches Page NO-22	Keto pork chops with blue-cheese sauce Page NO- 49	Classic keto steak tartare Page NO- 66
Friday	Scrambled eggs Page NO- 23	Keto Thai fish curry and bok choy Page NO- 55	Broccoli cheddar soup 1/3 of amount Page NO- 72
Saturday	Scrambled eggs Page NO-23	Beef patties with creamy onion gravy Page NO- 50	Classic keto steak tartare Page NO- 66

35-Days Keto Diet Weight Loss Challenge

Third Week Meal Plan

DAYS	BREAKFAST	LUNCH	DINNER
Sunday	Butter "bulletproof" coffee Page NO-30	Keto zucchini and walnut salad Page NO- 51	Seafood salad with avocado Page NO- 64
Monday	Scrambled eggs Page NO-23	Keto zucchini and walnut salad Page NO- 51	Keto oven-baked Brie Cheese Page NO- 64
Tuesday	Keto egg muffins Page NO-34	Keto fried salmon with Asparagus Page NO- 40	Keto harvest pumpkin and sausage soup Page NO- 66
Wednesday	Keto porridge Page NO-23	Keto tuna salad with poached eggs Page NO- 57	Classic keto steak tartare Page NO- 66
Thursday	Butter "bulletproof" coffee Page NO-30	1/2 amount of Keto salmon pie Page NO- 52	1/2 amount as serving: Spicy shrimp salad Page NO- 72
Friday	Low-carb chia pudding Page NO- 23	1/3 of the amount of Keto quesadillas Page NO- 52	1/2 amount of Keto pizza Page NO- 65
Saturday	Salad sandwiches Page NO-22	Keto fried halloumi cheese with mushrooms Page NO- 53	Keto tuna salad with poached eggs Page NO- 57

35-Days Keto Diet Weight Loss Challenge

Fourth Week Meal Plan

DAYS	BREAKFAST	LUNCH	DINNER
Sunday	1-minute keto mug muffins Page NO- 23	Keto chili bake Page NO- 63	Keto pork chops with asparagus Page NO-54
Monday	Butter "bulletproof" coffee Page NO-30	Avocado bacon and chicken bun-less burger Page NO- 53	Keto egg casserole with zucchini and ham Page NO- 54
Tuesday	1-minute keto mug muffins Page NO-23	Quick keto curry bowl Page NO- 54	Keto Thai fish curry and bok choy Page NO- 55
Wednesday	Keto meatloaf muffins Page NO-21	Loaded keto breakfast wrap Page NO- 22	Keto chilli bake Page NO- 53
Thursday	Loaded keto breakfast wrap Page NO-22	Keto pork chops with asparagus Page NO-54	Avocado bacon and chicken bun-less burger Page NO- 53
Friday	Keto meatloaf muffins Page NO-21	Keto egg casserole with zucchini and ham Page NO- 54	Quick keto curry bowl Page NO- 54
Saturday	Loaded keto breakfast wrap Page NO-22	Keto Thai fish curry and bok choy Page NO- 55	Steak with keto mushroom sauce Page NO- 67

35-Days Keto Diet Weight Loss Challenge

Fifth Week Meal Plan

DAYS	BREAKFAST	LUNCH	DINNER
Sunday	Butter "bulletproof" coffee Page NO-30	Keto salmon-filled avocados Page NO- 55	Keto turkey plate Page NO- 55
Monday	Keto breakfast tapas Page NO-22	Keto turkey plate Page NO- 55	Keto tuna and avocado salad Page NO- 55
Tuesday	Salad sandwiches Page NO-22	Keto tuna and avocado salad Page NO- 55	Italian plate Page NO- 56
Wednesday	Butter "bulletproof" coffee Page NO-30	Italian plate Page NO- 56	Salad Niçoise Page NO- 56
Thursday	Salad sandwiches Page NO-22	Salad Niçoise Page NO- 56	Keto roast beef and cheddar plate Page NO- 67
Friday	Keto breakfast tapas Page NO-22	Keto tuna salad with boiled eggs Page NO- 56	Classic keto steak tartare Page NO- 66
Saturday	Butter "bulletproof" coffee Page NO-30	Keto salmon-filled avocados Page NO- 55	Keto tuna plate Page NO- 68

BREAKFAST RECIPES

Keto Berry Bake

While we recommend having a good source of protein at your first meal, this recipe is a lovely treat on cold winter mornings. The berry bake can be eaten both hot and cold - we prefer it hard with a dollop of Greek-style yogurt.

Made for: Breakfast | **Prep Time:** 10 minutes | **Servings:** 4
Per Serving: Kcal: 265, Carbs 5.7g, Protein 6.6g, Fat 23.4g

Ingredient
- 250g Soft Cream Cheese (alternatives: Ricotta or Mascarpone)
- 175g Fresh Soured Cream (alternatives: Greek or Greek Style Yogurt or Creme Fraiche)
- 2 Large Eggs
- 15g Truvia / Natvia / Pure Via Sweetener
- 15ml Lemon Juice
- 1 tsp Vanilla Extract
- 100g Mixed Berries

Instructions
1. Preheat the oven to 180c.
2. If using a food processor/blender, all ingredients can be added simultaneously except the fruit and blended to a smooth paste.
3. If mixing by hand, combine the eggs, cream cheese, and sour cream in a large mixing bowl.
4. Add the lemon juice, sweetener, and vanilla extract.
5. Put the fruit into an ovenproof dish(es) and pour the mix over the fruit.
6. Bake for 30-40 minutes or until golden and the mix is firm.

Berry Chia Pot

Made for: Breakfast | **Prep Time:** 5 minutes | **Servings:** 2
Per Serving: Kcal: 131, Carbs 3.3g, Protein 5.7g, Fat 8.8g

Treat this like overnight oats - prepare it the night before for a refreshing breakfast. You could also add sweetener or vanilla essence if needed. Swap the frozen berries for 20g of cocoa powder to make a cocoa chia pot. You'll likely need to add some sweetness to this mix.

Ingredient
- 400ml Unsweetened Almond Milk
- 50g Frozen Berries
- 40g Whole or Milled Chia Seeds

Direction

1. Mix the ingredients, portion into dishes/jars, and allow to sit for a few hours - preferably overnight.
2. If the mix isn't enough for you, increase the chia seeds by 10g per portion.

Keto Chaffee

Some recipes call for adding almonds to help with stability, but we've decided to omit them as the crispy grated mozzarella seems to do that nicely.

Made for: Breakfast | **Prep Time:** 10 minutes | **Servings:** 4
Per Serving: Kcal:218, Carbs1.5g, Protein 18.4g, Fat 15g

Ingredients
- 75g Grated Mozzarella (pre-grated)
- 3 Large Eggs
- Spices & Seasoning to taste - e.g., Garlic Powder & Italian Herbs

Directions
1. Beat the eggs and add the grated mozzarella and spices/seasoning. Mix until thoroughly combined.
2. Pour half of the mix into the waffle press (use a quarter of the mix if you have a smaller waffle maker). Cook for 1-2 minutes until golden brown.

Cheese & Tomato Omelette

Made for: Breakfast | **Prep Time:** 5 minutes | **Servings:** 1
Per Serving: Kcal: 355, Carbs 4.6g, Protein 20.7g, Fat 28.5g

Ingredients
- 10g Butter
- 2 Large Eggs, whisked
- 50g Baby Cherry / Plum Tomatoes
- 30g Mature Cheddar, grated
- Handful of spinach
- Seasoning & spices to taste

Directions
1. Melt the butter on medium heat in a frying pan and add the tomatoes and spinach.
2. Cook for 3-5 minutes, and add the whisked eggs (mix any spices into the eggs before cooking).
3. As the eggs begin to firm, add the cheese on top.
4. Season and cook the omelette to your preference.

Cheesy Scrambled Eggs

Made for: Breakfast | **Prep Time:** 5 minutes | **Servings:** 1
Per Serving: Kcal: 345, Carbs (net) 2.5 grams, Protein 20.4 grams, Fat 28.4 grams

Ingredients
- 10g Butter
- 2 Large Free Range Eggs
- 30g Cheddar Cheese, grated
- 30g Spinach
- Salt & Pepper to taste

Directions
1. Melt the butter on medium heat in a large pan and add the eggs.
2. While stirring the eggs, add the cheese. You can also add the spinach here or place it on your plate if you prefer it fresh.
3. Cook the eggs to your preference and season.

Keto meatloaf muffins

This fun keto recipe will have skeptics asking for more of these delicious meatloaf muffins by Libby Jenkinson. The versatility of this recipe allows you to customize the muffins to your unique taste. Don't forget the cheese!

Made for: Breakfast | **Prep Time:** 5 minutes | **Servings:** 1
Per Serving: Kcal: 283, CARBS 2g, PROTEIN 26g, FAT 18g

Ingredients
- 1/6 (18 g) yellow onion diced finely
- 110 g ground beef or ground turkey
- 1/3 lightly beaten large egg
- 1/3 tbsp Italian seasoning
- salt and pepper to taste
- 20 ml (9 g) shredded mozzarella cheese
- 10 ml grated parmesan cheese (optional)

Instructions
1. Preheat the oven to 350°F (180°C).
2. Place the onion, meat, eggs, Italian seasoning, salt, and pepper in a large bowl.
3. Mix all the ingredients with your hands and place a small handful of the meatloaf mixture into muffin trays (2 per serving). Press gently; otherwise, they will turn into meatballs.
4. Cover with the grated cheese, and sprinkle with grated parmesan if desired. Cook in the oven for 20-30 minutes or until meat reaches 165°F (75°C).

Choco Waffles

A sight adaption to our nut-free fluffy pancakes mix, this recipe makes a great breakfast and a delicious dessert! Serve with Greek or Greek-Style yogurt, berries, almond butter, or even a drizzle of pouring cream :)

Made for: Breakfast | **Prep Time:** 5 minutes | **Servings:** 2
Per Serving: Kcal: 156, Carbs (net) 2.9 grams, Protein 11.2 grams, Fat 8.9 grams

Ingredients
- 4 Large Eggs
- 80ml Unsweetened Almond Milk (or other milk of your choice - e.g., cartooned coconut 'milk')
- 35g Coconut Flour
- 10g Cocoa Powder
- 25g Truvia / Natvia / Pure Via Sweetener
- 1 tsp Vanilla Essence / Extract
- 1/2 tsp Baking Powder

Directions
1. Whisk the eggs, milk, and vanilla together in a bowl.
2. Add the remaining ingredients and whisk until smooth.
3. Pour a third of the mix in a good non-stick pan, a crepe pan, or a waffle press. If you're cooking these in a pan, you may need to add around 5g of butter to the pan first and pour the mixture into smaller amounts to make lots of mini pancakes instead of a few large ones.
4. Allow the mix to cool until air bubbles appear on the top. Gently turn the pancake over to finish cooking. If you open your waffle press too early, the waffle may split in half!

Cinnamon Crunch

This lovely granola has a slightly 'lighter' texture than our original recipe... if that makes sense. Of course, the mixed spice/cinnamon isn't necessary, but it's a lovely addition!

Made for: Breakfast | **Prep Time:** 5 minutes | **Servings:** 10
Per Serving: Kcal: 97, Carbs (net) 1.7 grams, Protein 2.1 grams, Fat 8.7 grams

Ingredients
- 25g Unsalted Butter or Coconut Oil (Cooking Coconut Oil has no taste)
- 50g Coconut Chips / Flakes
- 30g Sunflower Seeds
- 30g Pumpkin Seeds
- 20g Whole Golden Linseed
- 10-15g Truvia / Natvia / Pure Via Sweetener

- 1/2 tsp Vanilla Extract
- 1/2 - 1 tsp Mixed Spice or Cinnamon (adjust to taste)

Directions
1. Preheat the oven to 180°C.
2. Melt the butter/coconut oil in the microwave or a small saucepan over gentle heat.
3. Add the melted butter/oil to a mixing bowl and all other ingredients and mix well to coat the seeds & coconut chips with the spice & sweetener. Adjust the sweetener to taste - we use very little as the coconut chips are pretty sweet.
4. Transfer the mix to an oven tray (if it's not very non-stick, line it with greaseproof baking paper or a silicone mat) and bake for around 10-15 minutes until golden. You may need to stir the mix halfway through baking to prevent the sides from burning.
5. Allow cooling before transferring to a storage container/jar. Keep in a cool cupboard (it'll last several weeks... although we eat it too quickly!).

Loaded keto breakfast wrap

Treat yourself to a hearty and healthy keto breakfast by Libby Jenkinson that will keep you full for hours. The classic breakfast flavors of bacon, cheese, and avocado form a hearty wrap to get your day started right. Check out the tips section below for various filling options that suit your inventory!

Made for: Breakfast | **Prep Time:** 5 minutes | **Servings:** 1
Per Serving: Kcal: 635, CARBS 4g, PROTEIN 28g, FAT 55g

Ingredients

Filling
- 28 g cooked bacon, chopped
- ¼ (50 g) avocado, diced
- 3 tbsp mozzarella cheese, shredded
- 1 tbsp sour cream

Wrap
- 2 eggs
- 2 tbsp heavy whipping cream
- salt and ground black pepper
- ½ tsp chili powder
- ½ tbsp fresh chives
- 1 tbsp butter

Instructions

Filling

1. Fry the bacon in a large frying pan over medium heat for 10 minutes or until crispy. Place bacon on paper towels to absorb excess fat. Once cooled, chop or cut into small pieces and set aside.

Wrap
2. Whisk the eggs, cream, chili powder, chives, salt, and pepper in a small bowl.
3. Melt the butter in the frying pan, then pour in the egg mixture.
4. Swirl the frying pan until the egg mixture is evenly spread and thin. This will act as the wrap for your filling.
5. Place a lid over the egg 'wrap' and leave to cook for 2 minutes.
6. Gently lift the egg 'wrap' from the frying pan with a clean spatula onto a plate.
7. Fold mozzarella cheese, bacon, avocado, and sour cream in the egg wrap. Enjoy!

Keto breakfast tapas

Made for: Breakfast | **Prep Time:** 5 minutes | **Servings:** 2
Per Serving: Kcal: 478, CARBS 6g, PROTEIN 24g, FAT 39g

Ingredients
- 55 g (120 ml) cheddar cheese
- 110 g prosciutto
- 110 g chorizo
- 2 tbsp mayonnaise or vegan mayonnaise
- 55 g cucumber
- 28 g (45 ml) red bell peppers

Instructions
1. Cut the cold cuts, cheese, and vegetables into sticks or cubes.
2. Arrange on a plate, serve and enjoy.

Salad sandwiches

Made for: Breakfast | **Prep Time:** 5 minutes | **Servings:** 2
Per Serving: Kcal: 472, CARBS 5g, PROTEIN 11g, FAT 44g

Ingredients
- 110 g (550 ml) Romaine lettuce or baby gem lettuce
- 4 tbsp mayonnaise
- 55 g (120 ml) Edam cheese or other cheese of your liking
- 1 (200 g) avocado, sliced
- 8 (140 g) cherry tomatoes, sliced

Instructions
1. Rinse the lettuce thoroughly and use it as a base for the toppings.
2. Spread butter or mayonnaise on the lettuce leaves, and layer the cheese, avocado, and tomato. Enjoy!

Scrambled eggs

Made for: Breakfast | **Prep Time:** 5 minutes | **Servings:** 2
Per Serving: Kcal: 415, CARBS 1g, PROTEIN 19g, FAT 37g

Ingredients
- 4 tbsp butter
- 6 large eggs
- salt and pepper

Instructions
1. Crack the eggs into a small bowl and use a fork to whisk them together with some salt and pepper.
2. Melt the butter in a non-stick skillet over medium heat. Watch carefully — the butter shouldn't turn brown!
3. Pour the eggs into the skillet and stir for 1–2 minutes, until they are creamy and cooked just the way you like them. Remember that the eggs will still be cooking even after putting them on your plate.

Keto porridge

Made for: Breakfast | **Prep Time:** 5 minutes | **Servings:** 2
Per Serving: Kcal: 644, CARBS 5g, PROTEIN 12g, FAT 64g

Ingredients
- 2 tbsp chia seeds
- 2 tbsp sesame seeds
- 2 eggs
- 160 ml heavy whipping cream
- 2 pinches salt
- 55 g butter or coconut oil

Instructions
1. Mix the chia seeds, sesame seeds, egg, heavy whipping cream, and salt in a medium-sized bowl. Set aside for 2–3 minutes.
2. Heat the olive oil or butter (until melted) in a small pan over medium heat.
3. Add the seed mixture, and stir together for about 2-3 minutes, or until the porridge thickens.
4. Top with the melted butter for serving, or perhaps with our low-carb raspberry jam.

Low-carb chia pudding

Made for: Breakfast | **Prep Time:** 5 minutes | **Servings:** 2
Per Serving: Kcal: 568, CARBS 8g, PROTEIN 9g, FAT 56g

Ingredients

- 475 ml unsweetened, canned coconut milk or unsweetened almond milk
- 4 tbsp chia seeds
- 1 tsp vanilla extract

Instructions
1. Mix all of the ingredients in a glass bowl or jar. Mix well.
2. Cover, place in the fridge to let gel overnight (or for at least 4 hours). Before you dig in, check to be sure the pudding has thickened and the chia seeds have gelled.
3. Serve the pudding with cream, coconut milk, or fresh or frozen berries.

1-minute keto mug muffins

Made for: Breakfast | **Prep Time:** 5 minutes | **Servings:** 2
Per Serving: Kcal: 329, CARBS 5g, PROTEIN 18g, FAT 25g

Ingredients
- 4 tsp butter or coconut oil for greasing
- 4 eggs
- 8 tsp coconut flour
- 1 tsp baking powder
- 2 pinches salt
- 8 tbsp feta cheese, crumbled or shredded cheddar cheese
- 4 tbsp fresh basil, roughly chopped

Instructions
1. For each serving, grease one ramekin or large coffee mug with butter.
2. Combine the egg, coconut flour, baking powder, and salt in a bowl. Mix well with a whisk or fork. Allow the batter to thicken for a couple of minutes.
3. Add the feta cheese and basil. Stir until combined.
4. Spoon the batter into the ramekins or microwave-safe mugs. Cook in the microwave on high for 45 seconds to one minute. Alternatively, these can be baked at 400°F (200°C) for 12 minutes.
5. Let the muffins cool before eating.

Coconut & Linseed Porridge

Made for: Breakfast | **Prep Time:** 5 minutes | **Servings:** 2
Per Serving: Kcal: 149, Carbs (net) 3.5 grams, Protein 6.8 grams, Fat 9.3 grams

Ingredients
- 360ml/g Unsweetened Dairy-Free Milk (e.g., Almond, Coconut - carton not tinned, Hemp)
- 30g Coconut Flour
- 30g Milled Linseed

- Truvia / Natvia / Pure Via Sweetener to taste

Topping Suggestions

- Almond / Peanut Butter
- Berries
- Greek / Greek-Style Yogurt

Directions
1. Heat the milk in a saucepan.
2. Using a whisk, carefully mix the remaining ingredients into the milk.
3. Allow to heat through, but no need to bring it to boil. Heat until it is at your preferred consistency.
4. Serve with your chosen toppings!

Coconut Milk and Chia Seed Mousse

The coconut and chia seed mousse is one of Mark's favorite recipes and can be ready in less than 5 minutes. The chia seeds act as a thickener, binding the coconut milk to create a mousse. Any low-carb berries can be used to add some flavor, and sweeteners can be mixed in to taste. However, while this is an excellent source of fat, it is relatively low in protein - this isn't a problem if you top up your protein with your other meals.

Made for: Breakfast | **Prep Time:** 5 minutes | **Servings:** 2
Per Serving: Kcal: 248, Carbs (net) 6.2 grams, Fat 22.9 grams, Protein 2.1 grams

Ingredients
- 400g Coconut Milk (Tinned)
- 25g Chia Seeds
- 100g Fresh or Frozen Berries - Raspberries, Blackberries, Strawberries
- Sweetener to taste - Truvia / Natvia / Pure Via

Directions
1. Mix all of the ingredients in a large bowl
2. Taste the mix and add any sweetener if required - add only 1/2 tsp at a time or a couple of Flavadrops
3. Divide into four equal portions and place in the fridge to thicken
4. Store in the refrigerator for up to 3 days.

Cooked Breakfast

Made for: Breakfast | **Prep Time:** 10 minutes | **Servings:** 1
Per Serving: Kcal: 394, Carbs (net) 3 grams, Protein 21.2 grams, Fat 32.1 grams

Ingredients

- 2 Rashers of Bacon
- 60g (1/2 medium) Avocado
- 1 Large Egg
- 70g Closed Cup Mushrooms
- 30g Spinach
- 10g Butter or Cooking Coconut Oil

Directions
1. Melt the butter/oil on medium heat and fry the bacon in a large pan.
2. Add the mushrooms.
3. If the pan is big enough, add the Egg and sliced avocado once the bacon is almost cooked. If not, wait until it is fully cooked, remove the bacon & mushrooms from the pan, and keep them warm while cooking your Egg and avocado.
4. Cook the egg to your preference and lightly brown the avocado.
5. Serve on a bed of spinach.

Pancakes (Crepes)

Thank you, Sara Goddard & Sue Chafer, for this recipe :-) The batter is very runny, but trust the process, and you will love them!

Made for: Breakfast | **Prep Time:** 5 minutes | **Servings:** 4
Per Serving: Kcal: 147, Carbs (net) 7.1 grams, Fat 11.2 grams, Protein 3.7 grams

Ingredients
- 60ml Double Cream
- 60ml Your favourite milk (I used Full fat Lactose-Free)
- 2 eggs
- 15g Arrowroot Powder
- Sweeten to taste - optional (leave the sweetener out for a savoury crepe)

Directions
1. Put all the ingredients in a food blender or a bowl and whisk till smooth
2. Get your suitable nonstick pan hot, with a bit of oil if needed
3. Pour a quarter into your pan and carefully spread it out thin
4. Cook for approx 30 - 60 seconds
5. Flip over and do the same on the other side

Classic bacon and eggs

One of the all-time best keto breakfasts ever! Step up your keto bacon and eggs game with this classic recipe. Gauge your hunger meter and enjoy as many eggs as you need to feel satisfied. We're drooling just thinking about this plate of keto deliciousness!

Made for: Breakfast | **Prep Time:** 5 minutes | **Servings:** 1
Per Serving: Kcal: 443, CARBS 2g, PROTEIN3 4g, FAT 32g

Ingredients
- 2 large eggs
- 65 g bacon, in slices
- cherry tomatoes (optional)
- fresh thyme (optional)

Instructions
1. Fry the bacon in a pan on medium-high heat until crispy. Put aside on a plate. Leave the rendered fat in the pan.
2. Use the same pan to fry the eggs. Place it over medium heat and crack your eggs into the bacon grease. You can also break them into a measuring cup and carefully pour them into the pan to avoid hot oil splattering.
3. Cook the eggs any way you like them. Leave the eggs to fry on one side for sunny side up, and cover the pan with a lid to make sure they get cooked on top. For eggs cooked over easy — flip the eggs over after a few minutes and cook for another minute. Cut the cherry tomatoes in half and fry them at the same time.
4. Salt and pepper to taste.

Keto Fluffy Waffles

Made for: Breakfast | **Prep Time:** 5 minutes | **Servings:** 3
Per Serving: Kcal: 201, Carbs (net) 3.9 grams, Protein 11.6 grams, Fat 13.7 grams

Ingredients
- 80ml/g Unsweetened Almond Milk (or other milk of your choice)
- 30g Coconut Flour
- 40g Ground Almonds
- 30g Truvia / Natvia / Pure Via Sweetener (adjust to taste)
- 3 Large Eggs
- 1/2 tsp Baking Powder
- 1/2 tsp Vanilla Extract
- Optional: 25g 85% Dark Chocolate

Directions
1. Combine the eggs and milk first, then add the remaining ingredients. If adding the chocolate, chop it up into tiny chunks and add it to the mix.
2. If using a waffle maker, add a third of the mix (or less if your waffle maker is small) and cook for around 3 minutes until golden.
3. If using a pan, add some butter if it's prone to sticking. Pour one portion into the pan and heat - to start, make several smaller pancakes. Allow cooking until air bubbles begin to appear in the top. Gently turn the pancake over to finish cooking.

Nut-Free Fluffy Pancakes

These can be batch-cooked and stored in the fridge or freezer, or the mix can be stored in the refrigerator for a couple of days. Stir the mixture before cooking - you may need to add a dash of milk if the mix is thick.

Made for: Breakfast | **Prep Time:** 10 minutes | **Servings:** 3
Per Serving: Kcal: 150, Carbs (net) 2.8 grams, Protein 10.9 grams, Fat 8.2 grams

Ingredients
- 80ml/g Nut-Free Milk, e.g., Coconut (carton, not tinned) or Hemp
- 45g Coconut Flour
- 4 Large Eggs
- 25g Truvia / Natvia / Pure Via Sweetener
- 1/2 tsp Vanilla Extract
- 1/2 tsp Baking Powder
- Optional: 25g 85% Dark Chocolate

Directions
1. Combine the eggs and milk first, then add the remaining ingredients. If adding the chocolate, chop it up into tiny chunks and add it to the mix.
2. If using a waffle maker, add a third of the mix (or less if your waffle maker is small) and cook for around 3 minutes until golden.
3. If using a pan, add some butter if it's prone to sticking. Pour one portion into the pan and heat - to start, make several smaller pancakes. Allow cooking until air bubbles begin to appear in the top. Gently turn the pancake over to finish cooking.

Keto Granola

Made for: Breakfast | **Prep Time:** 10 minutes | **Servings:** 10
Per Serving: Kcal 105, Carbs (net) 0.8 grams, Protein 2.2 grams, Fat 10.1 grams

Ingredients
- 100g Nuts of your choice (e.g., Almonds, Pecans, Brazil Nuts, Hazelnuts)
- 45g Milled Linseed (or other milled nuts/seeds)
- 15g Flaked Almonds
- 25g Coconut Oil or Unsalted Butter
- 20g Truvia / Natvia / Pure Via Sweetener

Directions
1. Preheat the oven to 180°C.
2. Roughly chop the nuts of your choice (except the flaked almonds) in a food processor or by hand. You still want some chunks to give the granola a crunch.
3. Add the nuts to a mixing bowl and the seeds, flaked almonds, and sweeteners.
4. Melt the coconut oil or butter in the microwave and add this to your dry ingredients. Mix to coat the nuts and seeds in the oil.
5. Spread the granola mixture onto a baking tray lined with greaseproof paper (or a silicone mat) and bake for about 10 minutes or until golden brown. Be careful - they'll burn quickly!

Ham & Cheese Omelette

Made for: Breakfast | **Prep Time:** 5 minutes | **Servings:** 1
Per Serving: Kcal: 459, Carbs (net) 3.7 grams, Protein 33.2 grams, Fat 35.1 grams

Ingredients
- 10g Butter
- 3 Large Eggs, whisked
- 40g Cooked Ham (cubed or sliced)
- 30g Mature Cheddar, grated
- Seasoning/spices to taste (garlic and paprika work nicely)
- Handful of spinach

Directions
1. In a frying pan, melt the butter on medium heat and add the beaten eggs (mix any seasonings & spices into the eggs before cooking).
2. As the eggs start to cook, add the ham.
3. Sprinkle the cheese on top and cook the omelette to your preference.
4. Serve on a bed of spinach.

Hash Browns (Cheesy or Corned Beef)

Made for: Breakfast | **Prep Time:** 10 minutes | **Servings:** 4
Per Serving: Kcal: 121, 3.2g Carbs, 8.9g Protein, 6.6g Fat,

Ingredients
- 200g White Cabbage - Raw
- 100g Corned Beef or Grated Cheese (we use mozzarella)
- 1 Large Egg
- 25g Shallot or Leek
- 10g Psyllium Husks
- If frying: 20ml Olive Oil or Cooking Coconut Oil

Directions
1. If you're baking these, preheat the oven to 200°C.
2. These are best made using a food processor but can also be caused by hand. Using the chopping (S-shaped) blade, blitz the cabbage first and add the rest of the ingredients except the oil. Blitz again to combine. If making these by hand, finely chop everything and mix with the Egg in a bowl. If you're making the cheesy hash browns, you may need to add an extra egg to get the mix to hold together.
3. If frying, add the oil to a pan over medium heat.
4. Using damp hands, mold the mix into oval patties and add to the pan or place on an oven tray lined with greaseproof baking paper.
5. Frying: Allow them to cook for 3-5 minutes before turning them over using a spatula. Allow cooking for a further 5 minutes. They will firm up during the cooking process but handle them carefully, so they don't break.
6. Baking: Cook for 10-15 minutes until firm and golden, then flip them over and bake for another 5 minutes to get them crispy on the other side :)

Keto Ketobix

Made for: Breakfast | **Prep Time:** 10 minutes | **Servings:** 20
Per Serving: Kcal: 65, 0.6g Carbs, 1.3g Protein, 6g Fat

Ingredients
- 50g Mixed Nuts
- 50g Mixed Seeds
- 50g POTATO FIBRE
- Pinch Salt
- 20g Ground Chia seeds
- 10g Truvia / Natvia / Pure Via Sweetener

- 100g Melted butter
- 100ml Water

Directions
1. Oven 120C, Ninja Grill Dehydrate 90C, Ninja Foodie Bake 110C

2. Grind the mixed nuts, mixed seeds, and chia seeds to a fine powder
3. Put all the dry ingredients into a large bowl and mix
4. Add the water and melted butter to the bowl and mix. It should look like damp sand....almost the texture of sand when you are about to build a sandcastle :-) * If your seed mix is linseed dominated, add a little more water, maybe 10-20g more
5. Let it rest for 5 minutes
6. Press into your desired shapes; I used a falafel maker and made them no more than 1cm thick (if you go more comprehensive, you will need to extend your cooking time
7. Transfer to a lined Baking tray
8. Cook at 120C, for approx 1 hour, maybe a little more. We are drying out the biscuits, not cooking - This is important. When you snap one in half, if it looks moist, it cooks for a little longer
9. If you are cooking in the Ninja foodie, cook at 110C for approx.1 hour, or in the Ninja Grill, on Dehydrate at 90C for 2 to 2 1/2 hours

Linseed & Chia Porridge

Made for: Breakfast | **Prep Time:** 5 minutes | **Servings:** 2
Per Serving: Kcal: 168, Carbs (net) 1.5 grams, Protein 8 grams, Fat 12.4 grams

Ingredients
- 400ml/g Unsweetened Dairy-Free Milk (e.g., Almond, Coconut - carton not tinned, Hemp)
- 30g Milled Linseed
- 30g Chia Seeds
- Truvia / Natvia / Pure Via Sweetener to taste

Topping Suggestions
- Almond / Peanut Butter
- Berries
- Greek / Greek-Style Yogurt

Directions
1. Heat the milk in a saucepan.
2. Using a whisk, carefully mix the remaining ingredients into the milk.
3. Bring the milk to a boil.
4. Reduce the heat and allow it to simmer for 2-3 minutes until it is your preferred consistency.

Pork Breakfast Burgers

We use these instead of store-bought sausages in a fry-up or make breakfast wraps using the Cheesy Wraps mix. We served these with the cheesy wraps & Sandie's Ketchup in the photo.

Made for: Breakfast | **Prep Time:** 5 minutes | **Servings:** 4
Per Serving: Kcal: 160, Carbs (net) 0.1 grams, Protein 17 grams, Fat 10.2 grams

Ingredients
- 500g Pork Mince
- 1 Large Egg
- Seasoning to taste - we like to add garlic, paprika, and Italian herbs.
- 10ml Olive Oil or Coconut Oil or Lard

Directions
1. In a large bowl, break the mince apart.
2. Crack the egg into the bowl and add the Seasoning.
3. Thoroughly combine the mixture.
4. Form 6 burgers with damp hands. If you have a burger press, line both sides of the media with a circle of greaseproof paper and press the mince into shape.
5. Add the oil to the pan and, over medium heat, fry the burgers for 5-6 minutes on each side.

Keto Savoury Muffins

Made for: Breakfast | **Prep Time:** 5 minutes | **Servings:** 3
Per Serving: Kcal: 161, 2g Carbs, 7g Protein, 14g Fat, 1g Fibre

Ingredients
- 15g Butter
- 120g Soured Cream
- 3 Large Eggs
- 80g Ground Almonds
- 10g Coconut Flour
- 1 tsp Baking Powder
- Seasoning (salt, pepper, herbs & Kashmiri chilli)
- 2 Sausages (97% pork or Ketoroma), cooked & sliced into discs

Directions
1. Preheat the oven to 190°C.
2. Melt the butter and add to a mixing bowl and the soured cream. Could you give it a quick mix, then add the eggs? Mix again.
3. Now add the ground almonds, coconut flour, baking powder & Seasoning, and mix.

4. Add around 20g of the mixture to each silicone cupcake case.
5. Add a slice of the sausage in the center of each case and then divide the rest of the mix between the points to cover the link.
6. Bake for 10-15 minutes until golden & firm.

Keto Savoury Waffles

These are an excellent option for an on-the-go meal. Add chopped meat, veg, and any herbs & spices (this especially helps if making a waffle to bulk out the mix).

Made for: Breakfast | **Prep Time:** 5 minutes | **Servings:** 2
Per Serving: Kcal: 245, Carbs (net) 2.6 grams, Protein 11.4 grams, Fat 20.5 grams

Ingredients
- 30g Ground Almonds
- 2 Large Eggs
- 60g Soft Cream Cheese
- Seasoning & Spices to taste
- If using a waffle maker: 1/2 tsp Baking Powder

Directions
1. Using a Nutri-bullet / blender, mix all ingredients to create a smooth paste. You can also combine this by hand.

Waffles
1. Pre-heat your waffle maker and pour some of the mixes in - ours fits half of the mixture. Close the waffle maker and allow it to cook for a few minutes. Be patient - if the waffle splits when you open the press, it's been opened too early.

Pancakes
1. We recommend making mini pancakes as these are easier to handle. Place a few spoons of mix in a good non-stick frying pan or crepe pan and cook over medium heat. If your pan isn't as non-stick as it used to be, add a dash of butter or cooking coconut oil.
2. When tiny bubbles appear on the surface, carefully flip the pancake over and cook for another 30 seconds.

Bacon Cheeseburger Pie

Made for: Breakfast | **Prep Time:** 15 minutes | **Servings:** 4
Per Serving: Kcal: 531, Carbs (net) 1.3 grams, Protein 49.4 grams, Fat 37 grams

Ingredients
- 500g Minced Beef (approx. 15% fat)
- 4 Rashers Smoked Bacon

- 120g Soured Cream
- 20g Lard / Olive Oil
- 6 Large Eggs
- 100g Mature Cheddar Cheese
- 1/2 tsp Onion or Garlic Powder
- 1/2 tsp Mixed Herbs

Directions
1. Preheat the oven to 180°C.
2. Cut the bacon into pieces.
3. In a non-stick frying pan, fry the bacon and beef mince together until all the beef mince has browned.
4. Add the seasonings to the pan.
5. Transfer the cooked meat into an ovenproof dish.
6. In a bowl, mix the eggs with the soured cream. Pour over the top of the meat and sprinkle the grated cheese.
7. Bake for 20-25 minutes or until the mix is firm on top.

Beef & Tomato Meatloaf

Made for: Breakfast | **Prep Time:** 10 minutes | **Servings:** 4
Per Serving: Kcal: 426, 4.8g Carbs, 64.4g Protein, 16.2g Fat

Ingredients
- 750g Beef Mince (5% Fat)
- 100g Shallots, diced
- 1 Large Egg
- 75-100g 'Breadcrumbs' - make a 90-second bread or use any other low-carb bread, like our Linseed Bread recipe or Mega Loaf.
- 1 tsp Dried Thyme
- 1 tsp Garlic Powder or 2-3 Garlic Cloves, finely chopped
- 100g Tomato Passata or Homemade Tomato Sauce
- 10ml Worcestershire Sauce
- Salt and Pepper to season
- Optional: 100g Pizza Mozzarella (in a block), sliced into thin strips

Directions
1. Preheat the oven to 180°C.
2. Put the beef mince in a large bowl and spend a minute kneading the meat.
3. Create a well in the meat and add all the other ingredients except 25g passata and (if you're using it) the mozzarella.
4. Thoroughly combine all the ingredients - this is best done by hand - and place the mix in a medium loaf tin (ours is 8.5" x 4").

5. Firmly press the mix into the loaf pan. If you're using the mozzarella, split the meat mix in half, press half into the bottom of the pan, and then layer the mozzarella slices in. Press the rest of the meat on top.
6. Bake for 30 minutes.
7. Spoon the remaining passata over the loaf and return to the oven for 10-15 minutes to finish cooking.
8. Allow resting for 10-15 minutes before slicing.

Chunky Beef Chilli

Made for: Breakfast | **Prep Time:** 10 minutes | **Servings:** 4
Per Serving: Kcal: 372, Carbs (net) 7.4 grams, Protein 35.7 grams, Fat 22.3 grams

Ingredients

- 40ml Olive Oil
- 80g Shallots
- 600g Diced Beef
- 200g Aubergine
- 80g Red Pepper
- 1 Beef Stock Cube in 200ml boiling water (if you're using a slow cooker, leave the stock cube as it is - sees instructions at the end of the method)
- 400g (1 tin) Chopped Tomatoes
- 1 Medium Hot Chilli or 1/2 tsp Chilli Flakes
- 2 tsp Garam Masala
- 1/2 tsp Ground Cumin
- Optional: 100g Soured Cream

Directions

1. Heat the oil in a large pan or wok over medium heat. Dice or slice the shallots and add them to the pan. Fry for 2-3 minutes until soft (not brown).
2. Turn the heat to high and add the diced beef. Cook on high until the meat has been browned on all sides.
3. Slice or dice the aubergine and pepper and add these to the pan. Cook for 1-2 minutes on high heat.
4. Add the beef stock and bring it back to boil.
5. Stir in the chopped tomatoes and spiced, return to boil, then reduce the heat to allow the dish to simmer for 45-60 minutes.
6. Season and stir in the soured cream when ready to serve.
7. In a slow cooker:

8. Follow steps 1-3, and then transfer to your slow cooker. Crumble a stock cube over the dish without the water and add the tomatoes and spices. Allow cooking for 6-8 hours on low. Season and add the soured cream when ready to serve.

Hash Browns (Cheesy or Corned Beef)

Made for: Breakfast | **Prep Time:** 10 minutes | **Servings:** 4
Per Serving: Kcal: 121, 3.2g Carbs, 8.9g Protein, 6.6g Fat

Ingredients

- 200g White Cabbage - Raw
- 100g Corned Beef or Grated Cheese (we use mozzarella)
- 1 Large Egg
- 25g Shallot or Leek
- 10g Psyllium Husks
- If frying: 20ml Olive Oil or Cooking Coconut Oil

Directions

1. If you're baking these, preheat the oven to 200°C.
2. These are best made using a food processor but can also be caused by hand. Using the chopping (S-shaped) blade, blitz the cabbage first and add the rest of the ingredients except the oil. Blitz again to combine. If making these by hand, finely chop everything and mix with the Egg in a bowl. If you're making the cheesy hash browns, you may need to add an extra egg to get the mix to hold together.
3. If frying, add the oil to a pan over medium heat.
4. Using damp hands, mold the mix into oval patties and add to the pan or place on an oven tray lined with greaseproof baking paper.
5. Frying: Allow them to cook for 3-5 minutes before turning them over using a spatula. Allow cooking for a further 5 minutes. They will firm up during the cooking process but handle them carefully, so they don't break.
6. Baking: Cook for 10-15 minutes until firm and golden, then flip them over and bake for another 5 minutes to get them crispy on the other side :)

Keto Cottage Pie

Made for: Breakfast | **Prep Time:** 25 minutes | **Servings:** 4
Per Serving: Kcal: 351, Carbs (net) 9.8 grams, Protein 36 grams, Fat 19 grams

Ingredients
- 40g Butter
- 100g Leeks
- 200g Courgette
- 500g Minced Beef (5%)
- 1 Beef Stock Cube in 200ml Boiling Water
- 800g (1 medium head) Cauliflower Florets
- 1/2 tsp thyme
- 40g Soft Cream Cheese
- Seasoning to taste

Directions
1. Preheat the oven to 180°C.
2. Heat the butter in a large pan or wok over medium heat. Dice or slice the leek and add to the pan. Fry for 2-3 minutes until soft, not brown.
3. Add the diced courgettes and fry for 2-3 minutes.
4. Either remove the leek/courgettes from the pan or push them to the side. Add the minced beef.
5. Cook the beef until brown and combine with the leek/courgette.
6. Add the beef stock. Bring to boil, then reduce the heat to simmer uncovered.
7. Break the cauliflower into small florets. Boil for 8-10minutes in a separate pan and drain well. Return them to the pan and add the Seasoning and cream cheese. Mash them together.
8. Once the meat stock has reduced, transfer the mix to an ovenproof dish and top with the cauliflower mash.
9. Finish in the oven for 20-25 minutes to allow the mash to brown.
10. Serve with some fried kale... proper winter grub!

Butter "bulletproof" coffee

What is bulletproof coffee, you ask? Quite simply, it's coffee mixed with butter and oil to help you feel satiated, alert, and focused on starting your day. A few sips of this piping hot keto coffee emulsion, and you'll be ready to take on the world. This recipe shows you how to make bulletproof coffee right at home. Fill 'er up!

Made for: Breakfast | **Prep Time:** 2 minutes | **Servings:** 1
Per Serving: 327, CARBS 0g, PROTEIN 1g, FAT 37g

Ingredients

- 240 ml hot coffee freshly brewed
- 2 tbsp unsalted butter
- 1 tbsp MCT oil or coconut oil

Instructions
1. Combine all ingredients in a blender. Blend until smooth and frothy.
2. Serve immediately.

Spiced Up Beef Burgers

Made for: Breakfast | **Prep Time:** 10 minutes | **Servings:** 4
Per Serving: Kcal: 262, 2.5g Carbs, 26g Protein, 16g Fat

Ingredients
- 20g Butter or Olive Oil
- 100g Shallots, finely chopped if not using a food processor
- 100g Red Pepper, finely chopped if not using a food processor
- 500g Aberdeen Angus Beef Mince (steak mince, 5-10% fat)
- 1 tsp Hot Chilli Powder
- 2 tsp Garam Masala
- Salt & Pepper to taste

Directions
1. Heat the butter/oil in a medium pan and fry the shallots & pepper over gentle heat for 6-8 minutes to slowly brown. Remove from the heat and allow to cool a little.
2. The burger mix can be made in a food processor or mixed by hand. Add all ingredients to a bowl/food processor and mix well.
3. Divide the mix into 4 or 8, depending on how thick you want each burger.
4. Use a burger press or mold the mix in your hands, pressing firmly.
5. Heat a skillet pan or a good non-stick frying pan over medium heat. Depending on the thickness of the burgers, fry for around 3-5 minutes on each side to ensure they are fully cooked.

Steak & Kidney Puddings

Made for: Breakfast | **Prep Time:** 10 minutes | **Servings:** 4
Per Serving: Kcal: 329, Carbs (net) 2.2 grams, Protein 44 grams, Fat 13.6 grams

Ingredients
- 20g Lard / Tallow
- 100g Shallots or Leeks, finely sliced
- 400g Shin Beef / Stewing Beef, diced
- 200g Lambs Kidneys
- 200ml Bone Broth / Bovril Cube
- 3-4 Sprigs of Fresh Thyme or 1 tsp Dried Thyme
- 1/2 tsp Salt
- Suet Pastry (see recipe)

Directions

1. Wash and prepare the kidneys (if they're not ready already) by removing the membrane and the tricky fatty bit in the middle of the kidney.
2. Heat the lard/fat in a large frying pan and gently fry the shallots for 2-3 minutes.
3. Add the beef & kidneys and fry for 3-4 minutes until brown.
4. Place the meat/shallots in the slow cooker and put the pan back on the heat. Add the stock to the pan to lift any meat/shallots off the pan, quickly bring it to the boil and pour it over the meat in the slow cooker.
5. Add the herbs & salt.
6. Allow the beef to cook covered on low for 6-8 hours. If you need to thicken the gravy, add a teaspoon of arrowroot powder to 20ml cold water, mix, and then add this to the slow cooker towards the end of the cooking process.
7. Use the Suet Pastry to line pudding tins and fill them with your slow cooker mix. Top it with a pastry lid and steam in a water bath for around 45 minutes.

Cheese in Blankets

Made for: Breakfast | **Prep Time:** 10 minutes | **Servings:** 4
Per Serving: Kcal: 165, Carbs (net) 0.3 grams, Protein 8.9 grams, Fat 12.7 grams

Ingredients
- 200g Halloumi or Grilling Cheese
- 8 Rashers of Streaky Bacon (smoked or unsmoked)

Directions
1. Cut the block of halloumi into 8 strips.
2. Wrap each piece in a rasher of bacon.
3. These can be cooked in a frying pan until the bacon is to your liking, or pop them in the air fryer for 10-15 minutes.

Cheese-Loaf & Burgers

Made for: Breakfast | **Prep Time:** 10 minutes | **Servings:** 4
Per Serving: Kcal: 484, Carbs (net) 5.9 grams, Protein 30.2 grams, Fat 36.5 grams

Ingredients
- 200g Halloumi / Grilling Cheese
- 50g Red Pepper, diced
- 50g Courgette, diced
- 25g Shallots / Leek, finely chopped
- 2 Large Eggs

- 10g Coconut Flour (alternatively, use 10g Psyllium Husk - see the description above for more details)
- 15g Chopped Fresh Herbs, e.g., Coriander, Thyme, Parsley
- 1/2 tsp Garlic Powder / Chilli Flakes / Smoked Paprika - you choose!

Directions
1. Preheat the oven to 180°C.
2. Blitz the halloumi/grilling cheese in a food processor to a fine crumb.
3. In a large bowl, combine all of the ingredients - you could do this in the food processor if you wanted finely diced veg, but don't over-process it as it will go watery.
4. Place the mix in a lined small loaf tin (ours is 9cm x 15cm) and bake for 30 minutes or until golden and firm. Or, divide the mix into little round dishes (2.5") and bake for 15 minutes.

Cheese-Slaw

Made for: Breakfast | **Prep Time:** 10 minutes | **Servings:** 4
Per Serving: Kcal: 118, 3g Carbs, 5.4 Protein, 8.8g Fat,

Ingredients
- 150g Hard White or Red Cabbage, thinly sliced
- 50g Carrot, thinly sliced
- 50g Leek, thinly sliced
- 50g Pepper, thinly sliced
- 50g Soured Cream
- 30g Creme Fraiche
- 100g Cheddar Cheese
- Salt, Pepper, and other spices/seasonings of choice

Directions
1. Add the chopped veg to a large mixing bowl.
2. Add the soured cream and creme fraiche to the bowl and stir to coat the veg. Add more of either soured cream or creme fraiche if you prefer a creamier coleslaw.
3. Finally, add the grated cheddar cheese and gently stir in the mix. Taste and add the seasonings of choice.

Cheese & Tomato Omelette

Made for: Breakfast | **Prep Time:** 5 minutes | **Servings:** 1
Per Serving: Kcal: 355, Carbs (net) 4.6 grams, Protein 20.7 grams, Fat 28.5 grams

Ingredients

- 10g Butter
- 2 Large Eggs, whisked
- 50g Baby Cherry / Plum Tomatoes
- 30g Mature Cheddar, grated
- Handful of spinach
- Seasoning & spices to taste

Directions
1. Melt the butter on medium heat in a frying pan and add the tomatoes and spinach.
2. Cook for 3-5 minutes, and add the whisked eggs (mix any spices into the eggs before cooking).
3. As the eggs begin to firm, add the cheese on top.
4. Season and cook the omelette to your preference.

Cheesy Wraps

Made for: Breakfast | **Prep Time**: 5 minutes | **Servings**: 4
Per Serving: Kcal: 263, 2g Carbs, 18.5g Protein, 19.9g Fat

Ingredients
- 250g Halloumi or Paneer or Mozzarella Ball (you could also use a mix of two or three)
- 5 Large Eggs

Suggested seasonings
- 1 tsp Garlic Powder + 1 tsp Italian Herbs
- 1 Small Bunch of Coriander, finely chopped + 1/2 tsp Ground Cumin
- 1/2 - 1 tsp Chilli Flakes + 1/2 - 1 tsp Paprika

Directions
1. Drain the water from the cheese and blitz it in a nutribullet / jug blender.
2. Add the eggs and blitz.
3. Divide into 5 equal portions (the mix will weigh around 500g so that each piece will be about 100g).
4. Fry in a good non-stick pan or crepe plate on low-medium heat for around 2 minutes. Leave the wrap alone until bubbles begin to form on the top! Flip and fry for approximately 30 seconds.

Goats Cheese Tart

Made for: Breakfast | **Prep Time**: 10 minutes | **Servings**: 4
Per Serving: Kcal: 517, Carbs (net) 4.9 grams, Protein 22.7 grams, Fat 43.8 grams

Ingredients

Pastry

- 100g Ground Almonds (or any other milled nuts or seeds, e.g., Milled Linseed)
- 1/4 tsp Xanthan Gum
- 25g Grated Parmesan
- 50g Butter, straight from the fridge and cut into small cubes
- 1 Large Egg
- 20g Coconut Flour

Topping
- 20g Butter
- 200g Leeks or Shallots, finely sliced
- 200g Goats Cheese
- 1 or 2 Sprigs of Fresh Thyme
- 50g Cherry Tomatoes, sliced

Directions
1. Preheat the oven to 180°C.
2. Add the ground almonds (or alternative), parmesan, and xanthan gum to a food processor and mix.
3. Add 25g of the butter, blitz for just a few seconds, then add the remaining butter and blitz again - the mix should now resemble large bread crumbs.
4. Add the egg and mix for 15-20 seconds, so the mix starts to form a dough.
5. Transfer this to another bowl and add the coconut flour. Mix using a spatula or a spoon - this will thicken the pastry.
6. Roll out the pastry between 2 sheets of greaseproof paper.
7. Line a non-stick oven-proof dish with the pastry (or separate the dough across little tartlet dishes) and gently press it into the sides of the word. It will break as you're doing this - don't worry; use spare pieces of dough to patchwork it back together.
8. Blind bake the pastry for 10 minutes.
9. Melt the butter in a pan and fry the leeks over medium heat until golden.
10. Once the pastry is cooked, spread the leeks on the base and lay the goat's cheese (and the cherry tomatoes if you're using them) on top. Sprinkle with the fresh thyme or your choice of fresh herb.
11. Bake for 15-20 minutes until golden brown.

Mini Cheddars

Made for: Breakfast | **Prep Time**: 25 minutes | **Servings**: 8
Per Serving: Kcal: 133, Carbs (net) 1 gram, Protein 7 grams, Fat 11 grams

Ingredients
- 25g Ground Almonds / Golden Linseed / Milled Mixed Seeds
- 175g Grated Cheddar Cheese

- 10g Grated Parmesan
- 30g Coconut Flour
- 1 tsp Mixed Herbs
- 1/2 tsp Garlic Powder
- 1/2 tsp Paprika
- 1/2 tsp Salt
- 1/2 tsp Pepper
- 30g Salted Butter, melted
- 1 Medium Egg

Directions

1. Preheat the oven to 180c
2. Melt the butter in the microwave and leave it to cool.
3. Add the ground almonds (or alternative), grated cheddar, parmesan, coconut flour, mixed herbs, garlic powder, paprika, salt, and pepper to a bowl and mix.
4. Then add the melted butter and Egg. Mix again.
5. Place the mix onto the worktop, form it into a dough, and knee it for a couple of minutes until smooth.
6. Divide into 5 or 6 pieces
7. Roll a piece between two sheets of greaseproof paper or silicone sheets. It will be very crumbly, but it molds together as soon as you start to roll it.
8. Roll the dough until it's about 3mm thick.
9. Using your cutter, cut out the mini cheddars. You could prick these with a fork to give it a nice effect.
10. The crackers are very fragile, so use a metal spatula to put them on the baking tray.
11. Cook on a lined tray for at least 10 minutes.
12. Adjust the time depending on your oven - mine took 15 minutes

Paneer & Coriander Fritters

Made for: Breakfast | **Prep Time:** 15 minutes | **Servings:** 3
Per Serving: Kcal: 262, Carbs (net) 4.7 grams, Protein 17 grams, Fat 19 grams

Ingredients

- 1 tsp Cumin Seeds
- 226g (1 block) Paneer Cheese
- 50g Spring Onions, finely sliced
- 2-3 Garlic Cloves, peeled & finely chopped
- 10g Fresh Ginger, peeled & finely chopped
- 10g Fresh Coriander
- 1/2 tsp Pink Himalayan / Rock / Sea Salt
- 2 Large Eggs
- 20g Coconut Flour

Directions

1. Heat a small frying pan over medium heat and, once hot, add the cumin seeds. You're only toasting these for 1-2 minutes - don't allow them to burn. Turn the heat off and set them aside while preparing the rest of the mix.
2. Break the paneer into small chunks and blitz in a food processor. If you don't have a processor, use a grater.
3. Add the finely chopped spring onions, garlic, ginger, coriander, cumin seeds, and salt to the food processor.
4. Start the processor and add the eggs to the mix. This process should only take 15-30 seconds. Don't over-process this, as you don't want a green paste!
5. Transfer the paneer mix into a bowl and add the coconut flour. Combine this and then divide the mixture into four portions.
6. From each portion, create 4 small balls, press them into shape and fry in a good non-stick frying pan over medium heat for 3-4 minutes on each side. Add some oil to the pan if needed.

Parmesan Rolls

Made for: Breakfast | **Prep Time:** 15 minutes | **Servings:** 4
Per Serving: Kcal: 225, Carbs (net) 2.3 grams, Protein 11.9 grams, Fat 18 grams

Ingredients

- 70g Grated Mozzarella or Mozzarella Block
- 30g Grated Parmesan plus 10g for topping
- 15g Psyllium Husks
- 100g Ground Almonds or other milled nuts/seeds (e.g., sunflower)
- 70g Milled Linseed
- 2 Large Eggs
- 100ml Cold Water
- 1.5 tsp Baking Powder
- 1 tsp Salt
- 1/4 tsp Garlic Powder
- Seasoning of your choice - we used dried mixed herbs

Directions

2. Preheat the oven to 180°C.
3. If you're using a mozzarella block, blitz this in a food processor until it resembles crumbs.
4. Add all the ingredients to 1 big bowl and stir well.
5. Allow the mix to rest for 5-10 minutes.

6. Using wet hands, separate the dough into rolls of equal weight. Place them a few centimeters apart on a lined baking tray.
7. If you're making filled rolls, mix the filling ingredients. Flatten each roll out in the palm of your hand and spoon some of the cream cheese into the center of the dough.
8. Carefully wrap the dough around the filling until it has all been concealed. Repeat for each dough ball and place them back on the tray.
9. Sprinkle the remaining 10g grated parmesan plus the garlic powder and any seasonings on top of the rolls.
10. Bake for 20-25 minutes until firm all around. They will be lovely and crispy on top! If they are going too brown on the outside, knock the temperature down to 160-170°C to ensure they're not doughy in the middle.

Tuna & Egg Salad

Made for: Breakfast | **Prep Time:** 10 minutes | **Servings:** 1
Per Serving: Kcal: 356, Carbs (net) 4.2 grams, Protein 39 grams, Fat 21 grams

Ingredients
- 120g (drained weight) Tinned Tuna in Spring Water - not oil
- 1 Large Hardboiled Eggs
- 15ml Olive Oil
- 30g Baby Spinach
- 50g Cherry Tomatoes
- 30g Cucumber

Directions
1. Boil, calm, and peel the Egg.
2. Chop up all ingredients, add to a bowl, and then drizzle with olive oil. Season to taste - simple!

Egg Fried Rice

Made for: Breakfast | **Prep Time:** 5 minutes | **Servings:** 2
Per Serving: Kcal: 428, 9.9g Carbs, 34.8g Protein, 25.3g Fat

Ingredients
- 500g Cauliflower / Broccoli (whole or as store-bought 'rice')
- 40g Unsalted Butter / Olive Oil
- 1 Small Bunch Spring Onions, finely chopped
- 100g Green Pepper or Broccoli Florets
- 2 Garlic Cloves / 10g Garlic Puree
- 10g Ginger Puree
- 2 Large Eggs

- Optional: 400g Raw King Prawns (cooked) or 300g Raw Chicken (either breast or thigh meat), cooked

Directions
1. Using a food processor, blitz the cauliflower/broccoli into the rice.
2. Heat the butter/oil in a large frying pan/wok over medium heat and add the spring onion, pepper (or broccoli florets), garlic, and ginger.
3. Cook over medium heat to soften for 2-3 minutes.
4. If you're using the prawns or chicken, add these now and combine.
5. Add the 'rice' and fry on high heat for 1-2 minutes. Combine all ingredients, reduce the heat to low, and cover the pan with a lid.
6. Cook for 3-5 minutes, and add a little water if needed to prevent the rice from sticking to the pan.
7. Crack the eggs directly over the rice and combine over high heat.
8. Continue to stir fry for 1-2 minutes to ensure the eggs are fully cooked.
9. Season and serve with some chopped coriander to finish the dish.

Keto Egg Muffins

Egg muffins are a great grab-and-go snack. The macros are calculated for the bacon and mushroom muffins, but try experimenting with different combinations!

Made for: Breakfast | **Prep Time:** 10 minutes | **Servings:** 8
Per Serving: Kcal: 114, Carbs (net) 0.6 grams, Protein 8.2 grams, Fat 8.9 grams

Ingredients
- 180g Button Mushrooms
- 4 Rashers of Bacon
- 20g Butter
- 6 Large Eggs
- 30g Soured Cream
- Alternative Combinations:
- Mushrooms & Peppers
- Stilton & Broccoli
- Asparagus & Bacon

Directions
1. Preheat the oven to 180°C.
2. Dice the mushrooms and cut the bacon into strips.
3. Add the butter to a pan over medium heat and fry the bacon & mushrooms. Cook for 5-8 minutes.

4. Once cooked, equally divide the mix between the cases. These are best made in either silicone cupcake cases/molds or a non-stick muffin tray.
5. Whisk the eggs and soured cream and fill each case equally.
6. Bake for 15-20 minutes. The muffins will sink while cooling down.

Keto Foo Yung

Made for: Breakfast | **Prep Time:** 10 minutes | **Servings:** 1
Per Serving: Kcal: 413, Carbs (net) 4.3 grams, Protein 40.1 grams, Fat 25.4 grams

Ingredients
- 100g Roast Pork / Chicken or 200g Raw King Prawns
- 3 Large Eggs
- 1/2 inch cube of Fresh Ginger (finely sliced) or 1/2 tsp Ginger Puree
- 50g Spring Onions
- 10ml Olive Oil / Coconut Oil
- Salt & Pepper to season

Directions
1. Heat the oil in a small/medium frying pan and gently fry the ginger and spring onions for 2-3 minutes.
2. Add the meat (if using raw prawns, fry these with the spring onions & ginger for 4-5 minutes).
3. Whisk the eggs in a mixing bowl or use a hand stick blender in a tall container to make them frothy.
4. Turn the heat up to high and pour in the egg mix. For the first 30-45 seconds, you want to keep the eggs moving so they don't stick to the pan.
5. Using a spatula, keep mixing the eggs and scraping the side and bottom of the pan to fold in the more cooked parts of the Egg. This will prevent having a pool of uncooked Eggs at the top.
6. Turn the heat down to low and cook for 2-3 minutes to ensure the dish is fully cooked.

Ham & Cheese Omelette

Made for: Breakfast | **Prep Time:** 5 minutes | **Servings:** 1
Per Serving: Kcal: 459, Carbs (net) 3.7 grams, Protein 33.2 grams, Fat 35.1 grams

Ingredients
- 10g Butter
- 3 Large Eggs, whisked
- 40g Cooked Ham (cubed or sliced)
- 30g Mature Cheddar, grated
- Seasoning/spices to taste (garlic and paprika work nicely)
- Handful of spinach

Directions
1. In a frying pan, melt the butter on medium heat and add the beaten eggs (mix any seasonings & spices into the eggs before cooking).
2. As the eggs start to cook, add the ham.
3. Sprinkle the cheese on top and cook the omelette to your preference.
4. Serve on a bed of spinach.

Pesto Eggs

Made for: Breakfast | **Prep Time:** 5 minutes | **Servings:** 1
Per Serving: Kcal: 231, 0.9 Carbs, 13.9g Protein, 18.7 Fat

Ingredients
- 2 Large Eggs
- One portion (around 10g) of Homemade Pesto.

Directions
1. Heat a small non-stick pan over gentle heat.
2. Add the pesto, spreading it around the pan with the back of a spoon.
3. Allow the pesto to heat gently (as it is made of olive oil, you want to keep it on low heat), then crack the eggs into the pan.
4. Fry the eggs to your preference (we cover the pan with a lid to help them cook on top).

Keto Scotch Eggs

Made for: Breakfast | **Prep Time:** 15 minutes | **Servings:** 4
Per Serving: Kcal: 262, Carbs (net) 1.3 grams, Protein 30 grams, Fat 14 grams

Ingredients
- 5 Hardboiled Eggs (medium is best, but large also works - the mince may split a little)
- 500g Pork Mince with 5% Fat can be replaced by any other mince (lean is best, e.g., turkey), or our Ketoroma 97% Pork Sausage Meat!
- 1 Large Egg
- 50g Golden Milled Linseed/Flaxseed (or replace this for ground pork scratchings!)
- Seasoning to taste - e.g., garlic, paprika, mixed herbs, chilli flakes, Kashmiri chilli, Curry Blend... the options are endless!

Directions

1. Preheat the oven to 200°C.
2. Boil, cool, and peel the eggs.
3. Mix the linseed with the Seasoning of your choice in a bowl.
4. Mix the minced pork with a few herbs and spices to suit your taste.
5. Divide the meat into 5 equal portions (around 100g per Egg) and wrap the Egg, completely covering it with the mince.
6. Roll the Egg in the linseed mix to cover the surface.
7. Bake at 200°C for around 20-25 minutes. The scotch eggs may split slightly while baking if you're using large eggs.
8. You can also fry these - see the video below for details!

Keto Shakshuka

Made for: Breakfast | **Prep Time:** 15 minutes | **Servings:** 4
Per Serving: Kcal: 421, Carbs (net) 8 grams, Protein 26 grams, Fat 32 grams

Ingredients

- 30ml Olive Oil
- 100g Shallots or Leeks, finely diced
- 3-4 Garlic Cloves, finely chopped (or 10g Garlic Paste)
- 60g Chorizo (replace this with 100g halloumi/grilling cheese for a vegetarian dish)
- 200g (an average) Courgette, finely diced
- 100g Green Pepper, finely diced
- 400g (1 tin) Chopped Tomatoes
- 2 tsp Smoked Paprika
- 1 tsp Ground Cumin
- 1/2 tsp Pink Himalayan / Rock / Sea Salt
- 1/2 tsp Chilli Flakes (optional)
- 8 Eggs
- 100g Grated Manchego Cheese

Directions

1. Preheat the oven to 190°C.
2. Heat the olive oil gently and add the shallots/leeks, garlic & chorizo (or halloumi).
3. Cook gently to soften the shallots for 2-3 minutes, turn the heat up, and add the courgette and pepper. Fry for 3-5 minutes, and then add the tin of chopped tomatoes plus half a can of water. Stir and bring to boil over medium / high heat.
4. Once up t the temperature, reduce the heat, add the spices and Seasoning, stir and cover. Allow cooking for 10-15 minutes over low heat.
5. Transfer the mix to a large oven-proof dish or into 4 individual plates and evenly spread the mixture.
6. Create dips in the mix and crack an egg so the yolk sits in the drop - the white of the Egg will sit on top.
7. Repeat for all eggs and pop in the oven for 15-20 minutes.
8. Remove from the oven, add the grated manchego and return to the oven for 5-10 minutes.

Baked Basa Fillet

Made for: Breakfast | **Prep Time:** 10 minutes | **Servings:** 1
Per Serving: Kcal: 456, Carbs (net) 11 grams, Protein 47.8 grams, Fat 26.1 grams

Ingredients

- 190g Basa Fillet (or Cod or Haddock fillets)
- 50g Leek or Spring Onions, finely sliced
- 50g Red / Yellow Peppers, finely sliced
- 100g Coconut Milk (as high % coconut extract as you can get) - can be swapped with Soured Cream or Greek / Greek-Style Yogurt
- 5ml Lemon Juice
- 1/2 tsp Ground Cumin
- 1 tsp Ground Coriander
- 1/2 tsp Ginger Puree
- 1/8 tsp (a pinch) Cayenne Pepper

Directions

1. Preheat the oven to 180°C.
2. Spread the peppers & leek/spring onions on the bottom of a small ovenproof dish.
3. Lay the fish fillet either in small strips or while fillet over the peppers & onions.
4. Mix the coconut milk, lemon juice, and spices and evenly spread them over the fish.
5. Cover the dish with foil and bake for 25-30 minutes.
6. E straight from the dish or use a spatula to lift from the container. Don't discard the excess liquid! Serve with low-carb veggies/salad and dress with infused juice.

Keto Fish Bites

Made for: Breakfast | **Prep Time:** 10 minutes | **Servings:** 2
Per Serving: Kcal: 495, 1.5g Carbs, 43.2g Protein, 34.7g Fat

Ingredients

- 375g Fresh Skinless Fish - Macros are for Skinless Cod
- 3 Large Eggs

- Coconut Oil / Lard for frying (500g-1kg, depending on the size of your pan)

Directions
1. Dice the fish and place it into a small food blender.
2. Add the eggs to the blender and any seasoning you choose - Our favourites are Smoked Paprika and Garlic (1/2 tsp of each) / 1 tsp Keto & Spice Curry Blend / 1/2 tsp, Dried Dill
3. Blitz the fish & eggs for 15 - 20 seconds. Don't over blend this - it should look like a lumpy paste.
4. Heat the oil in a large frying pan/wok to 190 degrees - use a thermometer to check the temperature.
5. Add a dessert spoon of the mix to the oil at a time once the oil is full to temperature. Don't add too many as this will reduce the temperature of the oil.
6. Cook for around 5 minutes or until the fish bites are cooked thoroughly - above 63 degrees.
7. Remove the bites from the oil and place absorbent paper to remove any excess oil.

Korma (Chicken, Halloumi, and Prawns)

Made for: Breakfast | **Prep Time:** 10 minutes | **Servings:** 4
Per Serving: Kcal: 413, 7.3g Carbs, 33.7g Protein, 27.1g Fat

Ingredients
- Proteins
- 400g Grilling Cheese / Halloumi OR 500g Raw Diced Chicken Breast OR 600g Raw King Prawns (fresh or frozen)
- 10ml Olive Oil
- 1 tsp Curry Blend
- 1 tsp Garam Masala

Sauce
- 80g Shallots, finely diced
- 1 tsp Garlic Puree
- 100ml Water
- 20ml Olive Oil
- 1 tsp Ginger Puree
- 1/2 tsp Ground Cumin
- 1/2 tsp Ground Coriander
- 1 tsp Turmeric
- 150g Tinned Coconut Milk (as high % coconut extract as you can find - Lidl is good for this)
- 100g Soured Cream / Greek or Greek-Style Yogurt / more Coconut Milk
- 40g Ground Almonds

Directions

Proteins
1. If using frozen prawns, ensure these are fully defrosted before using them. If using chicken or halloumi, dice this into bite-sized pieces. Place your chosen protein in a mixing bowl.
2. Add the oil & spices and combine to coat the protein.
3. Once you have prepared the sauce, heat a large frying pan. Fry the chicken for around 8-10 minutes, the halloumi for 5 minutes, and the prawns for 3-4 minutes on medium / high heat.
4. Mix with the sauce and serve. If using chicken, ensure that it is fully cooked.

Sauce
1. To create a smooth korma sauce, we start with an onion & garlic paste. Put the diced onion and garlic in a small food processor/blender and add 100ml water. Blitz until you have a smooth paste.
2. Heat the olive oil in a medium frying pan and once the oil is hot, add the paste. It will spit and steam a fair amount, so be careful when pouring the paste in.
3. Fry the paste over medium heat until almost all of the liquid has cooked away.
4. Add the ginger and all the ground spices.
5. The mix will turn into a thick paste. Allow this to cook over low-medium heat for 3-5 minutes.
6. Add the coconut milk, soured Cream (or alternative), ground almonds, and stir.
7. If the sauce is too thick, add a little water to create your preferred consistency.

Salmon Terrine

Made for: Breakfast | **Prep Time:** 20 minutes | **Servings:** 8
Per Serving: Kcal: 342, 2.9g Carbs, 18g Protein, 29g Fat

Ingredients
- 400g Smoked Salmon - if you're making 1 large taurine, you won't need as much. 300g will be more than enough
- 250g Cream Cheese
- 100g Very soft butter, but not liquid. My kitchen was particularly cold, so I gave it a quick blast in the microwave
- 150g Cooked Salmon - flaked into very small pieces
- 100g Cucumber - skinned & finely chopped - These are for the filling
- 120g Cucumber - skinned & very finely sliced - these are for the base
- Whole lemon zest
- 1 tbsp lemon juice, approx half lemon juice

- 2 tsp wholegrain mustard or horseradish - both are delicious
- 2 Tbsp Chives - finely chopped
- Salt & Pepper - season to taste
- 1 Tbsp Dill for decoration
- Some lemon slices to decorate

Directions

1. Lightly oil your tin or ramekins with oil (water will work as well) & then line it with clingfilm. Make sure there is plenty of cling film hanging over the outside of your ramekins or tin
2. Grind black pepper into the base of the clingfilm-lined tin or ramekins. then place your lemon slices and finally break off pieces of dill and place them in the base or bases
3. If you're doing individual ramekins, it's 50g of smoked salmon per ramekin. Completely line your dishes/tin with the slices of smoked salmon. Allow the salmon to drape over the outside

The Filling

1. Add to a food processor - Cream Cheese, softened butter, lemon zest & lemon juice & whiz till smooth
2. Transfer to a large bowl
3. Now add all the other ingredients - flaked salmon, 100g finely chopped cucumber, whole grain mustard or horseradish, finely chopped chives
4. Mix well, taste now season with salt & pepper & mix again
5. Compact it well into your dishes, and then put your finely sliced cucumber over the top, completely sealing the filling
6. Fold the remaining lost bits of smoked salmon over the top of the cucumber. If it completely seals the cucumber, great; if not, that's fine too :-)
7. Now seal the dish with the overhanging clingfilm
8. With your hands, gently compact it into the dish/dishes and chill for a couple of hours.
9. So long as all the ingredients are fresh, this will keep in the fridge for a few days
10. To turn out of the dish/dishes, open up the clingfilm, pop a plate on top, and turn it upside down, et voila!
11. Enjoy

Salmon Wellington

Made for: Breakfast | **Prep Time:** 20 minutes | **Servings:** 4
Per Serving: Kcal: 620, Carbs (net) 4.4 grams, Fat 49 grams, Protein 38 grams

Ingredients

- 4 x 120g Salmon Fillets
- 100g Baby Leaf Spinach
- 60g Mascarpone Cheese
- 100g Ground Almonds or Milled Seeds (e.g., milled linseed)
- 50g Butter
- 1 Large Egg
- 20g Coconut Flour
- 25g Grated Parmesan
- 1/4 tsp Xanthan Gum

Directions

1. Firstly make the pastry. Using a small food processor, add the ground almonds, parmesan, and xanthan gum and mix for a couple of seconds.
2. Add 25g of the butter and blitz for a few seconds.
3. Repeat the step with the remaining butter. The mix should now resemble bread crumbs.
4. Add the egg and mix for 15-20 seconds, so the mix starts to form a dough but doesn't overmix.
5. Transfer the mix to another bowl and add the coconut flour. Mix using a spatula or spoon - this will thicken the pastry.
6. If you are making individual portions, separate the dough into 4 equal portions and roll each out between 2 sheets of greaseproof paper to around 15 cm round / 6 inches.
7. Using a frying pan with a well-fitting lid, wilt the spinach over medium / low heat (you may need to add a little water to start the spinach to wilt.
8. Once the spinach has wilted, add the mascarpone cheese and cook over low heat until the mascarpone is fully combined with the spinach.
9. Allow the spinach to cool a little before making the parcels.
10. Using one piece of pastry, lay a salmon fillet in the center, add a small amount of wilted spinach and evenly spread along the fillet. Sprinkle with any herbs and Seasoning before sealing the pastry.
11. Using the greaseproof, bring in the pastry to wrap the fillet. Use the paper to help you press the pastry in place.
12. Transfer the fillets to a baking tray and bake at 180c for 20 - 25 minutes.
13. For a larger fillet, bake for an extra 10 minutes.

LUNCH RECIPES

Keto Fiery Wings

Made for: Lunch | **Prep Time:** 10 minutes | **Servings:** 4
Per Serving: Kcal: 633, Carbs (net) 2.1 grams, Protein 60.6 grams, Fat 44.7 grams

Ingredients
- 1kg Chicken Wings
- 30ml Olive Oil
- 2 Whole Red / Green Chillies, finely sliced
- 2 Garlic Cloves or 5g Garlic Puree
- 20g Fresh Coriander
- 2 tsp Kashmiri Chilli

Directions
2. If you want a smooth paste to coat the chicken, blitz the oil, chilies, garlic, and coriander in a small food processor or, if you're feeling energetic, use a pestle & mortar to grind it into a smooth paste. If you prefer to have pieces of chilli and garlic, finely chop these along with the coriander and mix with the oil & spices.
3. You can separate the joints of the wings by running a knife between the joints or leaving them whole. Place the wings in a zip-lock food bag and pour over the marinade.
4. Remove any air and seal the bag. Carefully massage the marinade into the wings and leave it in the fridge overnight.
5. Layer them in your air fryer or on a baking tray and cook at 200°C for 20-25 minutes or to your preference.

Battered Chicken

Made for: Lunch | **Prep Time:** 10 minutes | **Servings:** 4
Per Serving: Kcal: 371, Carbs (net) 3.7 grams, Protein 59.9 grams, Fat 12.7 grams

Ingredients
- 600g Chicken Breast
- 60g Ground Almonds (this recipe works better if the almonds are very fine - blitz them in a Nutri-bullet to do this)
- 60g Vital Wheat Gluten or Egg White Protein + another 30g for dipping in
- 2 tsp Baking Powder
- 2 Large Eggs
- 1/4 tsp Salt
- 200ml Sparkling Water
- Cooking Coconut Oil or lard for frying

Suggested additions:

- For southern-fried, use 1 heaped tsp Smoked Paprika, 1 tsp Garlic Powder, 1 tsp Dried Thyme & 1 tsp Onion Powder.
- For a Chinese-style batter, add 1/2 tsp Ginger Powder, 1 tsp Garlic Powder, and 1 tsp Five-Spice Powder

Directions
1. Add the salt, ground almonds, 60g of the vital wheat gluten (or all of the egg white powder), and the baking powder to a mixing bowl. Mix. Add your seasonings if you wish here too.
2. Add the eggs and sparkling water and whisk well. Set aside for 10 minutes. The batter should be reasonably gloopy to ensure it sticks to the chicken.
3. Start your deep fat fryer heating to 180°C or heat your oil pan now.
4. Chop your chicken up into even-sized pieces. I got 8 good-sized pieces per breast.
5. Coat lightly, using the rest of the vital wheat gluten on a plate before dipping it into your batter. Allow the excess to drain before gently placing it into your hot oil.
6. Once the batter is a good color, flip the pieces over to ensure both sides are evenly cooked.
7. Cook until the chicken is 83°C inside, about 5-7 minutes. Make sure chicken is fully cooked before eating.
8. Drain the chicken pieces before eating.
9. If you don't have enough oil to deep fry, shallow fry the pieces long enough for the batter to set and turn golden. You will need to flip the pieces part way through to ensure they're golden.
10. We then placed the chicken in the air fryer and air-fried it for 10 minutes at 190°C to ensure the chicken was at 83°C inside. This also dries the batter a bit and gives you a nice crunch!

Butter Chicken Curry

Made for: Lunch | **Prep Time:** 10 minutes | **Servings:** 4
Per Serving: Kcal: 404, Carbs (net) 4.9 grams, Protein 38 grams, Fat 26 grams

Ingredients
- 600g Diced Chicken Breast
- 60g Butter or Ghee
- 80g Shallots
- 120g Fresh Tomatoes
- 2-3 Garlic Cloves
- 10g Ginger Puree
- 2 tsp Garam Masala

- 1/4 tsp Chilli Flakes
- A handful of fresh coriander, chopped, or 1 tsp chopped frozen coriander
- 200g Soured Cream

Directions

1. Place the chicken in a bowl/container big enough to mix in the marinade.
2. In a food processor / mini food chopper, add the coriander, onion, garlic, spices, soured cream, and puree in a food processor/mini food chopper.
3. Add the marinade mix to the chicken and stir thoroughly to cover all of the chicken. Leave for a minimum of 20 minutes or preferably overnight.
4. Heat the butter in a large pan or wok over medium heat.
5. Roughly chop the tomatoes (we used cherry tomatoes, so cut them in half) and add them to the butter. Allow them to cook over gentle heat for around 5 minutes.
6. Over medium heat, add the chicken pieces and slowly cook for 5 minutes, then start to turn the pieces over to ensure the chicken is cooked thoroughly on both sides.
7. Allow the chicken to cook for at least 12-15 minutes over a very gentle heat - make sure it doesn't dry out. Add the rest of the marinade in while it's cooking.

Keto fried salmon with asparagus

Made for: Lunch | **Prep Time:** 5 minutes | **Servings:** 1
Per Serving: Kcal: 591, NET CARBS 2g, PROTEIN 28g, FAT 52g

Ingredients
- 110 g green asparagus
- 45 g butter
- 130 g salmon, boneless fillets, in pieces
- salt and pepper

Instructions
1. Rinse and trim the asparagus.
2. Heat a hearty dollop of butter in a frying pan where you can fit both the fish and vegetables.
3. Fry the asparagus over medium heat for 3-4 minutes. Season with salt and pepper. Gather everything in one half of the frying pan.
4. If necessary, add more butter and fry the pieces of salmon for a couple of minutes on each side. Stir the asparagus now and then, and lower the heat towards the end.

5. Season the salmon and serve with the remaining butter.

Cajun Chicken

Made for: Lunch | **Prep Time:** 5 minutes | **Servings:** 2
Per Serving: Kcal: 272, Carbs (net) 4.8 grams, Protein 37.5 grams, Fat 11.5 grams

Ingredients
- 20ml Olive Oil / 20g Butter
- 50g Shallots, finely chopped
- 2 Garlic Cloves, finely chopped or 1 tsp Garlic Puree
- 1 tsp Paprika
- 1/4 tsp Cayenne Pepper
- 1/2 tsp Dried Thyme
- 300g Chicken Breast - Raw & Sliced
- 100g Red Peppers, finely sliced
- Salt & Pepper to taste
- Optional: Chilli Flakes

Directions
1. Heat the oil gently in a large frying pan and fry the shallots and garlic for 1-2 minutes.
2. Keep the heat low and add the paprika, cayenne pepper, and dried thyme. Combine this with the oil & onions.
3. Lay the chicken pieces over the top of the onions, cover with a lid and allow to cook for 3-5 minutes.
4. Turn the chicken over and add the strips of pepper. Cover again and cook for a further 3-5 minutes.
5. Remove the lid, turn the heat up to medium/high, and quick fry everything together.

Chicken & Avocado Salad

Made for: Lunch | **Prep Time:** 5 minutes | **Servings:** 1
Per Serving: Kcal: 346, Carbs (net) 1.2 grams, Protein 24.3 grams, Fat 26.8 grams

Ingredients
- 100g Diced Chicken Breast
- 1/2 (around 60g) Avocado, sliced
- 15ml Olive Oil
- Handful of spinach

Directions
1. Heat the oil in a frying pan/wok over gentle heat.
2. Add the chicken and brown it on all sides. Allow cooking over medium heat for 5 minutes.

3. Move the chicken to the side of the pan and add the avocado.
4. Handle the avocado gently and fry until golden on all sides.
5. Serve on a bed of spinach.

Keto Caesar salad

A true keto salad classic: moist chicken and crispy bacon are served on a bed of crunchy Romaine lettuce. We don't skimp on the dressing or the parmesan cheese in our version!

Made for: Lunch | **Prep Time:** 15 minutes | **Servings:** 1
Per Serving: Kcal: 1076, CARBS5g, PROTEIN64g, FAT87g

Ingredients

Dressing
- 60 ml mayonnaise
- ½ tbsp Dijon mustard
- ¼ lemon, zest, and juice
- 30 ml (10 g) grated shredded Parmesan cheese
- 1 tbsp finely chopped filets of anchovies
- ½ garlic clove, pressed or finely chopped
- salt and pepper

Salad
- 170 g chicken breasts, bone-in with skin
- salt and pepper
- ½ tbsp olive oil
- 45 g bacon
- 100 g (500 ml) Romaine lettuce, chopped
- 60 ml (20 g) shredded Parmesan cheese

Instructions
1. Preheat the oven to 350°F (175°C).
2. Mix the ingredients for the dressing with a whisk or an immersion blender. Set aside in the refrigerator.
3. Place the chicken breasts in a greased baking dish.
4. Season the chicken with salt and pepper and drizzle olive oil or melted butter on top. Bake the chicken in the oven for about 20 minutes or until fully cooked. You can also cook the chicken on the stovetop if you prefer.
5. Fry the bacon until crisp. Place lettuce as a base on two plates. Top with sliced chicken and the crispy, crumbled bacon.
6. Finish with a generous dollop of dressing and a good grating of parmesan cheese.

Chicken, Bacon & Asparagus Salad

Made for: Lunch | **Prep Time:** 5 minutes | **Servings:** 1
Per Serving: Kcal: 341, Carbs (net) 1.8 grams, Protein 31.8 grams, Fat 23.6 grams

Ingredients
- 100g Chicken Breast
- 2 Rashers of Bacon
- 80g Asparagus
- Optional: 10g Parmesan Cheese, grated
- 15ml Olive Oil
- Handful of spinach

Directions
1. Heat the oil in a frying pan/wok over gentle heat.
2. Add the chicken and brown it on all sides. Allow cooking over medium heat for 5 minutes.
3. Move the chicken to the side of the pan and add the bacon. Fry for 1-2 minutes.
4. Add the asparagus.
5. Allow to cook for 2-3 minutes or until the asparagus is cooked to your taste.
6. Serve on a bed of spinach and serve with the parmesan cheese (optional).

Chicken & Chorizo

Made for: Lunch | **Prep Time:** 20 minutes | **Servings:** 4
Per Serving: Kcal: 563, 13g Carbs, 50.8g Protein, 33.6g Fat

Ingredients
- Follow the recipe for Rice Base Dish
- 20g Olive oil
- 400g Chicken breast - chunky chopped
- 250g Chorizo - chunky chopped
- 120g Red Pepper - chunky chopped
- 2 tsp Paprika
- 25g Fresh, flat-leaf parsley, roughly chopped
- Salt & pepper

Directions
1. Follow the instructions for the Rice Base Dish
2. Oven 180C, Ninja 170C, or this can be fried in a non-stick frying pan
3. Add chicken, chorizo, peppers, olive oil, paprika, and seasoning to a bowl. Could you give it a good mix?
4. Pop on the oven for about 25 - 30 minutes or until the chicken is cooked
5. Once cooked, add all the ingredients, including the fresh parsley, to the Rice Base recipe and stir through
6. This can be quickly stir-fried to reheat the rice dish or popped into the fridge

7. To reheat, either stir fry or microwave. If reheating in the oven, make sure you cover the dish with foil so it doesn't dry out
8. Enjoy :-)

Chicken Fritters

Made for: Lunch | **Prep Time:** 5 minutes | **Servings:** 2
Per Serving: Kcal: 337, Carbs (net) 4 grams, Protein 47 grams, Fat 15 grams

Ingredients
- 300g (approx. 2 average) Chicken Breast, raw - this could also be replaced with Turkey Breast
- 50g Grated Mozzarella
- 50g Soured Cream
- 10g Coconut Flour
- 1 Large Egg
- 1/2 tsp Salt
- Herbs / Spices to taste (we like to use garlic powder and a sprinkle of dried dill)

Directions
1. Slice the chicken breast into small strips and place in a large mixing bowl.
2. Add all of the remaining ingredients and mix well.
3. Heat a non-stick pan over medium heat - add 1 tsp cooking coconut oil if your pan isn't quite as non-stick as it used to be!
4. Take a heaped dessert spoon of the mix and pop it in the pan. You should get a nice sizzle but don't have the heat too high. We need the chicken to cook thoroughly inside without overcooking the outside.
5. Gently press the mix to flatten it a little and allow it to cook for 2 minutes.
6. Flip the cake over, gently press again and continue to cook for 2-3 minutes.
7. Each patty should take around 8-10 minutes to cook. If you're not sure, break one in half to check the meat is white all the way through.

Creamy Chicken & Ham Pie

Made for: Lunch | **Prep Time:** 10 minutes | **Servings:** 4
Per Serving: Kcal: 897, 9.1g Carbs, 51g Protein, 72g Fat

Ingredients
Pie Crust
- 1 batch Pie Crust (follow this link to take you to the recipe)

The Filling
- 400g Chicken - Small, roughly chopped

- 200g Cooked Ham or Gammon - Small, roughly chopped
- 300g Leeks - Small, roughly chopped
- 20g Butter
- 20g Olive oil
- 1/2 tsp garlic
- 250ml Milk
- 150ml Double Cream
- 1 Chicken stock cube
- 20g Parmesan
- 20g Arrowroot (mixed with about 30ml water to create a thickening agent)
- Salt & Pepper (I added 1/2 tsp salt & 1/4 tsp pepper)

Directions
Pie Crust
1. 1 batch Pie Crust (follow this link to take you to the recipe)

The Filling
1. Add the butter & Olive oil to a large pan and fry the leeks for about 5 - 10 minutes, until it's softened but not browned (almost translucent)
2. Now add the chicken & fry until cooked (about 5 - 10 minutes)
3. Add all the remaining ingredients APART from the arrowroot mixed with water, stir well and bring up to almost bubbling and turn down to a gentle simmer
4. Now add the arrowroot and stir through the sauce in the pan. Allow thickening. If you'd like it a little thicker, add more arrowroot, mixed with a little water in the same way. Or, if you'd like to keep the carbs lower, add a sprinkling of ready grated mozzarella & stir through until it thickens
5. Now pour into your prepared Pie Crust base and go back to the Pie Crust recipe and instruction no.8 onwards
6. Enjoy :-)

Keto Chicken Kyiv

Made for: Lunch | **Prep Time:** 10 minutes | **Servings:** 1
Per Serving: Kcal: 284, Carbs (net) 2.6 grams, Protein 44.7 grams, Fat 10.3 grams

Ingredients
- 180g (Medium / Large) Chicken Breast
- 1 Egg
- 20g Milled Golden Linseed
- 1/2 tsp Dried Mixed Herbs
- 30g Soft Cream Cheese
- 1 Garlic Clove (crushed) or 1/2 tsp Garlic Paste
- Salt & Pepper

Directions

1. Preheat either the oven or air fryer to 180°C.
2. Mix the egg in a big enough bowl to fit the chicken breast.
3. Mix the linseed with herbs & seasoning in another bowl (again, the bowl needs to be big enough for the chicken).
4. Slice the chicken breast in half length-ways, on the thickest side of the fillet. Be careful not to slice all the way through.
5. Mix the cream cheese and garlic in a small bowl. Spread the cream cheese on one side of the chicken fillet and fold the other side over.
6. Dip the chicken fillet into the egg and ensure that both sides are coated.
7. Lift the chicken from the egg mixture and allow any excess to drain off. Transfer the chicken to the linseed mix and coat both sides of the crumb again.
8. Place in a baking dish and pop in the oven for 25-30 minutes. Depending on the thickness of the fillet, it may require a little longer. To ensure it is fully cooked, pierce the chicken with a skewer - any liquid from the chicken should be clear.

Chicken, Leek & Broccoli Pie

Made for: Lunch | **Prep Time:** 15 minutes | **Servings:** 4
Per Serving: Kcal: 271, 3.8g Carbs, 32.8g Protein, 13.5g Fat

Ingredients
- 30ml Olive Oil or 30g Butter
- 500g Diced Chicken Breast (or swap this for Turkey Breast)
- 100g Leeks, finely sliced
- 200g Broccoli Florets
- 1 Vegetable / Chicken Stock Cube
- 100g Mascarpone Cheese or Soured Cream
- 1 tsp Dried Parsley or Mixed Herbs
- Pastry of choice - we use either the suet pastry or shortcrust pastry.

Directions
1. Preheat the oven to 180°C.
2. Heat the oil/butter over medium heat and add the chicken and leeks together. Fry for 3-5 minutes, turning the chicken to ensure all sides turn from pink to white.
3. Add the broccoli, combine everything in the pan, reduce the heat to low, and cover with a lid. Allow to cook for 5-8 minutes - this will allow the broccoli to soften and the chicken to fully cook.

4. There should be a little moisture in the pan from this part of the cooking process. If not, add around 50ml water and then crumble the stock cube over the mix. Ensure the stock cube is fully combined.
5. Replace the lid and allow to cook for 2-3 minutes.
6. Add the mascarpone cheese / soured cream and thyme. Stir to melt this through the dish.
7. Pour the mix into a pie dish.
8. Roll your pastry of choice between 2 sheets of greaseproof paper and place this over your pie filling. Bake for 25-30 minutes until the pastry is golden.

Chicken Stir Fry

Made for: Lunch | **Prep Time:** 10 minutes | **Servings:** 2
Per Serving: Kcal: 399, Carbs (net) 8.9 grams, Protein 39.1 grams, Fat 20.5 grams

Ingredients
- 30ml Olive Oil
- 300g Diced Chicken Breast
- 50g Mushrooms, sliced
- 50g Red Onion / Shallots, sliced
- 50g Carrot, sliced
- 100g White Cabbage, sliced
- 50g Bell Pepper, sliced
- 50g Courgette, sliced
- 1/2 tsp Garlic Puree
- 1/2 tsp Ginger Puree
- 1 tbsp Sesame Seeds

Directions
1. Heat the oil in a large pan and add the chicken. Fry for 2-3 minutes and turn to brown on all sides.
2. Add all of the sliced vegetables and fry for 1-2 minutes.
3. Add the garlic and ginger. Combine thoroughly.
4. Cover the pan with a lid and cook for 5 minutes over medium heat. If needed, add a little water to prevent the veg from sticking to the pan.
5. When you're ready to serve, season, sprinkle with sesame seeds, and enjoy :)

Chicken & Vegetable in Gravy Pie

Made for: Lunch | **Prep Time:** 15 minutes | **Servings:** 4
Per Serving: Kcal: 795, 7.6g Carbs, 50g Protein, 62g Fat

Ingredients
Pie Crust

- 1 batch Pie Crust (follow this link to take you to the recipe)

The Filling
- 600g Chicken - Small, roughly chopped
- 100g Swede - Small, roughly chopped
- 100g Leeks - Small, roughly chopped
- 100g Peppers - Small, roughly chopped
- 100g Celery - Small, roughly chopped
- 100g Mushrooms - Small, roughly chopped
- 50g Peas
- 40g Butter
- 100ml Double cream
- 2 Chicken stock cubes
- 300ml Boiling water
- 2 tsp Herbs
- 1/2 tsp Garlic
- Salt & Pepper (I added 1/2 tsp salt & 1/4 tsp pepper)

Directions
Pie Crust
1. 1 batch Pie Crust (follow this link to take you to the recipe)

The Filling
2. Pop the chopped-up swede in a microwave bowl with a little water and microwave for about 5 - 7 minutes. This is to speed up the cooking time of this vegetable, as the swede takes the longest to cook
3. Add the butter to a large pan and fry the leeks for about 5-10 minutes, until it's softened but not browned (almost translucent)
4. Now add the chicken & fry for a further 5 minutes
5. Add all the vegetables (apart from the peas) & the garlic and herbs and stir through and fry for a further 5 minutes
6. Add to the pan stock cubes, boiling water, and seasoning
7. Allow simmering for about 20 - 30 minutes, until all the vegetables are cooked
8. Add the cream & peas and stir through
9. If you'd like to thicken the sauce, either cook for a little longer or add some chia seeds, which act as a lovely thickening agent
10. Now pour into your prepared Pie Crust base and go back to the Pie Crust recipe and instruction no.8 onwards
11. Enjoy :-)

Chinese Vegetable Stir Fry

Made for: Lunch | **Prep Time:** 15 minutes | **Servings:** 2
Per Serving: Kcal: 149, Carbs (net) 8 grams, Protein 6 grams, Fat 10 grams

Ingredients
- 10ml Soy Sauce or Liquid Aminos
- 1/4 tsp Chilli Flakes
- 1 tsp Apple Cider Vinegar
- 100g Broccoli Florets, cut into small pieces
- 1 tbsp (15ml) Toasted Sesame Oil
- 80g (1 medium) Red Pepper, sliced into thin strips
- 100g (1 head) Pak Choi - remove the bottom 1-2 cm of the pak choi and slice thinly until you reach the dark leaf (see photo). Leave these unsliced to add to the dish at the very end.
- 2-3 Garlic Cloves, finely chopped
- 10g Peeled Fresh Ginger, finely chopped
- 50g (approx. 1 bunch) Spring Onions, thinly sliced
- 100g Beansprouts

Directions
1. In a small dish, mix the soy sauce / liquid aminos, chilli flakes, and apple cider vinegar - this will be used at the end of the cooking process.
2. Bring a pan of water to a boil, add a pinch of salt, and add the broccoli florets. Cook for 2-3 minutes. Remove from the heat, strain the water, and set aside.
3. Add the sesame oil to a frying pan over medium heat. Add the pepper and white strips of pak choi.
4. Cook for 2-3 minutes to soften, then add the garlic, ginger, spring onions, and broccoli.
5. Fry over medium heat for 3-5 minutes.
6. Turn the heat to high, add the beansprouts & green pak choi leaves, and pour over the liquid amino & chilli mix; quickly combine and serve.

Cock-a-Leekie Soup

Made for: Lunch | **Prep Time:** 15 minutes | **Servings:** 2
Per Serving: Kcal: 246, Carbs (net) 6.7 grams, Fat 13 grams, Protein 24.7 grams

Ingredients
- 500g Chicken Thighs, sliced into small chunks (approx. 2cm)
- 300g Leeks, sliced thinly

- 30g Soup & Broth Mix (This is the uncooked weight, and it's a mix of pearl barley, yellow and green split peas, marrowfat peas, and red split lentils) washed and drained
- 100g Carrots, Peeled and grated
- Well seasoned to taste

Directions
1. Add to a large pan all your ingredients
2. Add cold water, enough to generously cover all the ingredients
3. Bring to boil and then turn down to a simmer and pop the lid on
4. Make sure it doesn't boil dry and has plenty of fluid. Refer to the picture for how much liquid should be left :)
5. Let this gently simmer for about 1 hour, stirring occasionally

Coronation Chicken

Made for: Lunch | **Prep Time:** 10 minutes | **Servings:** 2
Per Serving: Kcal: 458, Carbs (net) 2.1 grams, Protein 32.6 grams, Fat 35.1 grams

Ingredients
- 250g Chicken Breast
- 1 tsp Ground Turmeric
- 1/2 tsp Salt
- 75g Rhubarb
- 1.5 tsp Truvia / Natvia / Pure Via Sweetener
- 10g Coriander, finely chopped
- 1/3 Red Pepper, finely chopped
- 2 Spring Onions, finely chopped
- 75g Mayonnaise (homemade or store-bought)
- 25g Greek or Greek Style Yogurt
- 1.5 tsp Curry Blend
- 10g Flaked Almonds
- 100g Romaine Lettuce

Directions
1. Cook the chicken breast in boiling water for around 15 minutes with turmeric & salt. Once the chicken is cooked, set it aside on a plate to cool down.
2. While the chicken is cooking, cut the rhubarb into small chunks. Cook in a pan with the sweetener and a little water for no longer than 2 minutes to retain some crunch. Set aside on a plate and let the rhubarb cool.
3. Add the remaining ingredients, except the almonds & lettuce, and mix in a bowl.

4. Chop the chicken into large cubes and add to the mix. Combine and taste for salt.
5. Add most of the rhubarb & flaked almonds to the bowl, holding some back for garnish. Fold in gently to prevent the almonds and rhubarb from breaking up.
6. Serve on a bed of lettuce leaves and garnish with the remaining almonds & rhubarb.

Crispy Coated Chicken Thighs

Made for: Lunch | **Prep Time:** 10 minutes | **Servings:** 8
Per Serving: Kcal: 315, Carbs (net) 1 gram, Protein 27 grams, Fat 22 grams

Ingredients
- 1kg / 8 average Chicken Thighs with skin and bone
- 50g Vital Wheat Gluten or Egg White Powder (we use this)
- 1 tsp Dried Oregano
- 1 tsp Paprika
- 1 tsp Garlic Powder
- 1 tsp Kashmiri Chilli
- 1/2 tsp Pink Himalayan / Rock / Sea Salt

Directions
6. Preheat the oven to 200°C or the Ninja Foodi (air crisp) / Air Fryer to 180°C.
7. In a large bowl, mix the vital wheat gluten with the spices & herbs. Reduce the chilli if you don't want these to be too spicy.
8. Flatten out the chicken thighs and place in the bowl (one at a time) with the spice/flour mix and fully coat. The chicken doesn't need to be dipped in egg first but is slightly wet to allow the coating to stick. The thighs are normally good to use straight from the packet, but if they've been opened and dried out of little, rinse them in a little cold water before adding them to the flour mix.
9. Lay the chicken thighs on a roasting tray and cook for 35-40 minutes. In a Ninja Foodi / Air Fryer, they may take less time.

Crunchy Chicken Bites

Made for: Lunch | **Prep Time:** 10 minutes | **Servings:** 6
Per Serving: Kcal: 208. 0.9g Carbs, 32.8g Protein, 8g Fat

Ingredients
- 85g Ready Grated Mozzarella
- 15g Cream Cheese
- 35g Ground Linseed or Ground Almonds

- 700g Chicken Breast, diced into bite-size chunks
- Seasoning of your choice, I put 1 tbsp of Curry Blend
- Salt and Pepper

Directions

1. Oven 180C
2. Put all the MKD ingredients into a microwave bowl
3. Microwave in 30-second blasts (normally a total of 90 seconds)
4. Mix with a spoon until a smooth dough ball forms
5. Roll out immediately on a sheet of greaseproof paper, put on an oven tray, and pop in the oven for 10 to 15 minutes, till nice and crispy
6. Leave the oven on while you do the next step until the chicken is ready to cook
7. Allow the MKD to cool. Add the cooled MKD to a bullet. Season well, add the Curry blend & Blitz till they resemble bread crumbs
8. Put the bread crumbs into a bowl. Start dunking your chicken into the bread crumbs, completely cover it
9. Lay these out onto a lined baking tray and pop into the oven for about 20 -25 minutes (until chicken is cooked)

Yogurt chicken kebabs with beet carpaccio

A rich curry and Greek yogurt-based marinade are key to these radiant and juicy, low-carb chicken kebabs. This tender combo is served with thinly sliced beetroots and tangy cilantro vinaigrette. Let it steal the spotlight at your next grill party!

Made for: Lunch | **Prep Time:** 20 minutes | **Servings:** 2
Per Serving: Kcal: 552, CARBS 9g, PROTEIN, 38g, FAT 39g

Ingredients
- 325 g boneless chicken thighs
- 60 ml (45 g) Greek yogurt (4% fat) or sour cream
- 1 tbsp curry powder or paprika powder
- ½ tbsp light olive oil
- ½ tsp salt
- ¼ tsp ground black pepper

Beet carpaccio
- 2 beets, red and yellow
- 45 g sugar snap peas
- ¼ (28 g) red onion, chopped

Cilantro vinaigrette
- 60 ml light olive oil
- 60 ml (4 g) fresh cilantro, chopped
- ½ tbsp lemon juice
- ½ garlic clove

- salt and ground black pepper

Instructions
1. Cut chicken into smaller pieces. Preheat the outdoor grill or oven with the grill function to 450°F (225°C).
2. Mix yogurt, curry, olive oil, pepper, and salt in a bowl. Cover chicken with marinade and let sit for at least 10 minutes. Place in the refrigerator overnight if you want to prepare the day before. Thread chicken pieces onto skewers just before you start grilling.
3. Scrub and rinse beets properly. Peel and cut into paper-thin slices, preferably with a mandolin. Remove strings from sugar snaps. Place vegetables and finely chopped onion on a plate.
4. Mix ingredients for vinaigrette with a hand blender. Drizzle over beet salad.
5. Grill chicken kebabs for 3-4 minutes on each side or until fully cooked and the inner temperature is 160°F (72°C).
6. Serve with beet carpaccio.

Curry Pasty Filling

Made for: Lunch | **Prep Time:** 20 minutes | **Servings:** 4
Per Serving: Kcal: 322, 8.5g Carbs, 17.2g Protein, 23.6g Fat

Ingredients
- 60g Chopped Swede
- 60g Chopped Celeriac
- 60g Chopped Leeks
- 15ml/g Olive Oil or Butter
- 1/2 tsp Salt
- 1/2 tsp Pepper
- 160g Chicken Breast (or 40g Lentils & 40g Chickpeas - uncooked weight)
- 30g Spinach
- 60g Sandie's Ketchup (or 30g Tomato Passata)
- 2 tsp Curry Blend
- 1 Garlic Clove or 1/2 tsp Garlic Powder
- 1 batch of MKD

Directions
1. Add oil or butter to the pan and heat up
2. Add all ingredients to the pan (if you're making the veggie curry, don't add the lentils and chickpeas just yet).
3. Slowly fry on low heat. Add a tiny bit of water to help the Swede cook. I added a tbsp at a time.
4. Keep cooking until the swede is almost cooked and the fluid has gone. You can now add the lentils & chickpeas (if you're using them) and stir.

5. Season to taste and allow to cool fully while you make the MKD.
6. Head to the MKD recipe to finish your pasties!

Keto Goan Curry

Made for: Lunch | **Prep Time:** 10 minutes | **Servings:** 4
Per Serving: Kcal: 493, 8.5g Carbs, 36.5g Protein, 34.2g Fat

Ingredients
- 150g Leeks / Shallots
- 30g Melted Butter or 30ml Olive Oil
- 4 Garlic Cloves
- 2 Fresh Red Chillies (this makes a mild sauce - increase to 4 for medium and 8 for a hot curry)
- 1 tsp Coriander Seeds
- 1 tsp Ground Turmeric
- 1/2 tsp Cumin Seeds
- 1/2 tsp Mustard Seeds
- 1 tbsp Tamarind Paste
- 400g Tinned Coconut Milk (as high % coconut as you can find - Lidl is good for this)
- 12 Large Hardboiled Eggs (this could be replaced with 600g (raw weight) Diced Chicken Breast, cooked)

Directions
1. Blend all ingredients except the tamarind paste, coconut milk, and eggs/chicken using a food processor. If the mix is too thick to blend, add 50-100ml water while blending.
2. Heat a large non-stick pan over medium heat and spread the paste around the pan to allow it to cook evenly. Keep the paste moving on medium / low heat.
3. After 2-3 minutes, add the tamarind paste, stir well, and add the coconut milk. Increase the heat to bring the sauce to a boil.
4. Add the eggs/chicken, stir well and then reduce the heat to low and cover.
5. Allow the dish to cook for a minimum of 15-20 minutes.

Hungarian Chicken

Made for: Lunch | **Prep Time:** 10 minutes | **Servings:** 4
Per Serving: Kcal: 334, Carbs (net) 4.5 grams, Protein 37.3 grams, Fat 18.2 grams

Ingredients
- 30ml Olive Oil
- 80g Shallots, thinly sliced
- 200g (1 medium) Courgette, thinly sliced
- 80g (1 medium) Red or Yellow Pepper, thinly sliced
- 2 Garlic Cloves, crushed or chopped
- 600g Diced Chicken Breast
- 1 tsp Paprika (smoked is best)
- 200g Soured Cream
- Salt & Pepper to taste

Directions
1. Heat 15ml of the oil over medium heat in a large pan or wok.
2. Once the oil is hot, add the onion, courgette, pepper, and garlic. Fry for 2-3 minutes until soft without browning,
3. Remove these from the pan and return the pan to the heat with the remaining oil.
4. Add the chicken pieces and brown on all sides.
5. Reduce the heat and cover the pan to allow the chicken to cook thoroughly for 8-10 minutes.
6. Add the paprika and return the vegetables to the pan.
7. Add the soured cream and combine.
8. Bring the sauce up to a boil and then reduce the temperature for 5-6 minutes.

Hunter's Chicken

Made for: Lunch | **Prep Time:** 10 minutes | **Servings:** 2
Per Serving: Kcal: 354, Carbs (net) 1.7 grams, Protein 42.4 grams, Fat 19.8 grams

Ingredients
- 240-300g (2 average) Chicken Breasts
- 4 Rashers of Smoked Back Bacon
- 4-6 tbsp Sandie's Ketchup
- 30g Mature Cheddar / Smoked Cheddar, grated
- 15ml Olive Oil
- A Pinch of Smoked Paprika
- 1 Pinch of Oregano
- Salt & Pepper

Directions
1. Preheat the oven to 190°C.
2. Butterfly the chicken by cutting through the breast, leaving a little hinge.
3. Cling film the breast and flatten each one evenly using a rolling pin or meat tenderizer.
4. Season what will be the inside of the chicken with salt & pepper.
5. Lay each chicken breast on rashers of bacon, spread a little of the ketchup on the chicken, and then roll the bacon & chicken with the bacon on the outside and the tomato on the inside.

6. Heat the oil in a frying pan and add each roll. Cook for 2-3 minutes to help seal the rolls and brown the bacon.
7. Place them in an ovenproof dish, add the remaining ketchup, sprinkle with paprika and oregano and cover with foil to bake for 15-20 minutes.
8. Remove the foil, sprinkle with cheese and bake for a further 10 minutes or until golden brown.

Kung Pao Chicken

Made for: Lunch | **Prep Time:** 10 minutes | **Servings:** 2
Per Serving: Kcal: 504, 8.5g Carbs, 35g Protein, 36g Fat

Ingredients
- 340g Chicken Thighs (skinless & boneless)
- 100g Courgette
- 100g Red Pepper
- 2 Tbsp Coconut Aminos (soy sauce alternative)
- 50g Peanuts (see description above for alternatives)
- 45ml Chicken Stock
- 60ml Olive Oil
- 20g Spring Onions
- 10g Toasted Sesame Oil
- 10g Truvia / Natvia / Pure Via Sweetener
- 10g Salt
- 2 Garlic Cloves
- 5g Thai Fish Sauce
- 5g Apple Cider Vinegar
- 2.5g Fresh Ginger
- 1/2 tsp Sesame Seeds
- 1/4 tsp Xanthan Gum
- 1/4 tsp Dried Red Chillies

Directions
1. In a medium bowl, combine all the ingredients for the sauce (chicken stock, coconut aminos, diced garlic, diced ginger). Set aside.
2. Season chicken with salt, pepper, and 1 tablespoon of sauce/marinade.
3. Add sesame & olive oil to a wok or a large non-stick skillet over medium-high heat.
4. Add the chicken and cook for 5-6 minutes, or until the chicken is starting to brown and almost cooked through.

5. Toss in the courgette, peppers, and dried chilli peppers (if using) and cook for 2-3 minutes, or until the vegetables are crisp-tender and the chicken is cooked through. Pour the remaining sauce and add the peanuts (slightly crushed up). Toss everything together and turn the heat to high. Allow sauce to reduce and thicken. Season with salt, pepper, or additional red pepper chilli flakes as needed, plus the sweetener (to taste). If desired, add 1/4 teaspoon xanthan gum to thicken the sauce further.
6. Remove from heat and serve warm on a large platter or over courgette noodles or cauliflower rice. Sprinkle with sesame seeds and spring onions if desired.

Chicken Moambe

Made for: Lunch | **Prep Time:** 10 minutes | **Servings:** 4
Per Serving: Kcal: 368, Carbs (net) 5.3 grams, Protein 41.9 grams, Fat 19.3 grams

Ingredients
- 600g Chicken Breast, diced
- 1 tsp Salt
- 1/2 tsp Cayenne Pepper / Hot Chilli Powder
- 1/2 tsp Ground Nutmeg OR 2 tsp Smoked Paprika (the nutmeg was the original recipe, but we have since updated this recipe to create a Winter Moambe using the paprika!)
- 250ml Water
- 15g Butter
- For the Winter Moambe, add 2 Garlic Cloves, finely chopped
- 150g Shallots, diced
- 1 Green Chilli, diced (and added to taste)
- 250g Tomato Passata or Tinned Chopped Tomatoes
- For the Winter Moambe: 1 tsp Bouillon / Vegetable Stock Cube
- 100g Peanut Butter or Almond Butter (100% nuts)

Directions
1. In a large saucepan, add the diced chilli and melt the butter.
2. Add the shallots (and garlic if you're using it) and fry for a couple of minutes to soften.
3. Add the chicken and cook until golden on all sides (around 10 minutes).
4. Add the passata (and, if you're using it, the bouillon/cube). Simmer for another 10 minutes, ensuring the chicken is fully cooked.

5. Turn off the heat and stir in the peanut/almond butter. If the butter is particularly thick (or cold), microwave it (in a microwavable container!) for just 15 seconds or so before stirring in.

Keto pork chops with blue-cheese sauce

Made for: Lunch | **Prep Time:** 10 minutes | **Servings:** 2
Per Serving: Kcal: 780, CARBS 4g, PROTEIN 54g, FAT, 60g

Ingredients
- 70 g blue cheese
- 90 ml heavy whipping cream
- 2 (550 g) pork chops
- salt and pepper
- 100 g fresh green beans
- 1 tbsp butter for frying

Instructions
1. Start by crumbling the cheese into a small pot over medium heat. Adjust heat as necessary to melt gently, and be careful not to let it burn. When the cheese has melted, add the cream and increase the heat slightly. Let simmer for a few minutes.
2. Season the chops with salt and pepper. Fry in a skillet on medium-high heat for 2-3 minutes before flipping. Cook until internal temperature is 145°-160°F (63°-71°C). Set aside and cover with foil for 2-3 minutes.
3. Pour the pan juices into the cheese sauce. Stir and, if needed, heat it again. As blue cheese is often fairly salty, taste the sauce before adding additional salt.
4. Trim and rinse the green beans. Fry them in butter for a few minutes on medium heat. Season with salt and pepper.

Keto ground beef and broccoli

Made for: Lunch | **Prep Time:** 10 minutes | **Servings:** 2
Per Serving: Kcal: 638, CARBS 5g, PROTEIN 47g, FAT, 46g

Ingredients
- 450 g ground beef or ground turkey
- 45 g butter or light olive oil
- 220 g (550 ml) broccoli
- salt and ground black pepper

Instructions
1. Rinse and trim the broccoli, including the stem. Cut into small florets. Peel the stem and cut it into small pieces.
2. Heat a dollop of butter in a frying pan where you can fit both the ground beef and broccoli.
3. Brown the ground beef on high heat until it is almost done. Season to taste with salt and pepper.
4. Lower the heat, add more butter, and fry the broccoli for 3-5 minutes. Stir the ground beef now and then.
5. Season the broccoli and serve while still hot.

Keto Caesar salad

Made for: Lunch | **Prep Time:** 10 minutes | **Servings:** 2
Per Serving: Kcal: 1076, CARBS 5g, PROTEIN 64g, FAT, 87g

Ingredients

Dressing
- 120 ml mayonnaise
- 1 tbsp Dijon mustard
- ½ lemon, zest, and juice
- 60 ml (20 g) grated shredded Parmesan cheese
- 2 tbsp finely chopped filets of anchovies
- 1 garlic clove, pressed or finely chopped
- salt and pepper

Salad
- 350 g chicken breasts, bone-in with skin
- salt and pepper
- 1 tbsp olive oil
- 85 g bacon
- 200 g (1 liter) Romaine lettuce, chopped
- 120 ml (40 g) shredded Parmesan cheese

Instructions
1. Preheat the oven to 350°F (175°C).
2. Mix the ingredients for the dressing with a whisk or an immersion blender. Set aside in the refrigerator.
3. Place the chicken breasts in a greased baking dish.
4. Season the chicken with salt and pepper and drizzle olive oil or melted butter on top. Bake the chicken in the oven for about 20 minutes or until fully cooked. You can also cook the chicken on the stovetop if you prefer.
5. Fry the bacon until crisp. Place lettuce as a base on two plates. Top with sliced chicken and the crispy, crumbled bacon.
6. Finish with a generous dollop of dressing and a good grating of parmesan cheese.

Keto chicken casserole

Made for: Lunch | **Prep Time:** 10 minutes | **Servings:** 2
Per Serving: Kcal: 617, CARBS 7g, PROTEIN 43g, FAT, 46g

Ingredients
- 60 ml heavy whipping cream
- 40 ml (40 g) cream cheese
- 1 tbsp green pesto
- 1/3 tbsp lemon juice
- salt and pepper
- 14 g butter
- 300 g skinless, boneless chicken thighs, cut into bite-sized pieces
- 55 g leeks, finely chopped
- 38 g cherry tomatoes, halved
- 110 g cauliflower, cut into small florets
- 160 ml (75 g) cheddar cheese, shredded

Instructions
1. Preheat the oven to 400°F (200°C).
2. Mix cream and cream cheese with pesto and lemon juice. Salt and pepper to taste.
3. In a large pan over medium-high heat, melt the butter. Add the chicken, season with salt and pepper, and fry until they turn golden brown.
4. Place the chicken in a greased 9 x 13" (23 x 33 cm) baking dish, and pour in the cream mixture.
5. Top chicken with leek, tomatoes, and cauliflower.
6. Sprinkle cheese on top and bake in the middle of the oven for at least 30 minutes or until the chicken is fully cooked. If the casserole is at risk of burning before it's done, cover it with aluminum foil, lower the heat, and let it cook for a little longer.

Beef patties with creamy onion gravy and broccoli

Made for: Lunch | **Prep Time:** 10 minutes | **Servings:** 2
Per Serving: Kcal: 880, CARBS 16g, PROTEIN 42g, FAT, 71g

Ingredients

Beef patties
- 325 g ground beef or ground turkey
- ½ egg
- 30 ml heavy whipping cream
- ½ (55 g) yellow onion, minced
- ½ tsp salt
- ¼ tsp ground black pepper
- 1½ tbsp butter

Onion gravy
- 1½ (170 g) yellow onions, thinly sliced
- 1 tbsp butter
- 160 ml heavy whipping cream
- ¼ tbsp tamari soy sauce
- salt and pepper
- Veggies
- 220 g (550 ml) broccoli or cauliflower

Instructions
1. Combine ground beef, egg, cream, minced onion, and the spices in a bowl. Use wet hands to form the flat patties.
2. Fry the patties in butter for 3-4 minutes on each side. Put the patties in an oven-proof dish and keep baking in the oven at 200°F (100°C) while you prepare the rest.
3. Whisk the cooking juices with some water and set aside for the gravy.
4. Slice the onions thin with a sharp knife or mandolin. Fry in butter until soft and golden. Set aside.
5. In a saucepan, bring the cream, cooking juices, and the rest of the ingredients for the sauce to a boil. Simmer over medium heat for 5-10 minutes or until the sauce has the desired consistency. Stir in the onions. Season with salt and pepper.
6. Rinse and cut the broccoli into smaller florets. Boil for a few minutes in lightly salted water until crisp-tender. Drain and allow to steam for a few minutes.
7. Serve the beef patties and the onion gravy with the freshly boiled broccoli.

Keto Tex-Mex burger plate

Made for: Lunch | **Prep Time:** 5 minutes | **Servings:** 2
Per Serving: Kcal: 828, CARBS 6g, PROTEIN 43g, FAT 68g

Ingredients
- 350 g ground beef or ground turkey
- 1 tbsp Tex-Mex seasoning or taco seasoning
- 2 tbsp olive oil
- salt and pepper
- 55 g (120 ml) sliced Pepper Jack cheese or Mexican cheese, or any other flavorful cheese you like
- 1 (200 g) avocado, sliced
- 55 g (350 ml) lettuce
- 2 tbsp pickled jalapeños, sliced
- 80 ml sour cream

Instructions
1. Mix ground beef and seasoning. Form one burger per serving.
2. Fry the burgers over medium heat, or grill, in half of the olive oil for 3-4 minutes until the burger is light pink or cooked through, whichever you prefer. Salt and pepper to taste.

3. Plate the burger and cheese, avocado, lettuce, jalapeños, and sour cream. Drizzle with the rest of the olive oil.

Pesto Kebabs

Made for: Lunch | **Prep Time:** 10 minutes | **Servings:** 4
Per Serving: Kcal: 578, 5.3g Carbs, 26.9 Protein, 50.3g Fat

Ingredients
- 1 batch of Pesto (also in OMG) - This can be made nut/dairy-free. See recipe for details.
- 4 Chicken Breasts (around 600g) / 400g Halloumi (100g per person).
- Juice of 1.5 Lemons (around 45ml)
- 200g of Bell Pepper (red, orange, or yellow)
- 200g Courgette
- Around 25g of Cherry Tomatoes (1 for each skewer)
- Steel or Wooden Skewers.

Directions
1. Preheat the oven to 220°C / Ninja Grill to High
2. If you're using wooden skewers, soak them in the water while prepping.
3. If you haven't already, make the pesto (in OMG).
4. Chop the chicken, pepper, and courgette into bite-size pieces/slices and add to a bowl with the pesto and lemon juice. Stir to cover everything.
5. Prepare your skewers, alternating between chicken and vegetables and skewering a cherry tomato on end for decoration 😀 .
6. Grill the kebabs for 26-20 minutes until the chicken is fully cooked. Part-way through baking, spoon over any remaining pesto mixture leftover in the bowl.

Keto turkey burgers with tomato butter

Made for: Lunch | **Prep Time:** 10 minutes | **Servings:** 1
Per Serving: Kcal: 783, CARBS 8g, PROTEIN 36g, FAT 67g

Ingredients

Chicken patties
- 170 g ground turkey or ground chicken
- ¼ egg
- 1/8 (14 g) yellow onion, grated or finely chopped
- ¼ tsp kosher or ground sea salt
- 1/8 tsp ground black pepper
- ¼ tsp dried thyme or crushed coriander seed
- 14 g butter, for frying

Fried cabbage
- 170 g green cabbage
- 21 g butter
- ¼ tsp salt
- 1/8 tsp ground black pepper

Whipped tomato butter
- 28 g butter
- ¼ tbsp tomato paste
- Tomato paste
- Also known as tomato puree
- ¼ tsp red wine vinegar (optional)
- sea salt and pepper to taste

Instructions
1. Preheat the oven to 220°F (100°C). Mix all ingredients for the patties in a bowl.
2. Shape the ground turkey into patties using wet hands. Fry in butter on medium-high heat until golden brown and fully cooked through. Place in the oven to keep warm.
3. Shred the cabbage using a sharp knife, mandolin slicer, or food processor.
4. Fry the cabbage in a generous amount of butter on medium-high heat until browned on the edges but still has somebody. Stir occasionally to make sure it cooks evenly. Season with salt and pepper. Lower the heat towards the end.
5. Place all ingredients for the tomato butter in a small bowl and whip them together using an electric hand mixer. Plate the turkey patties and fried cabbage and place a dollop of tomato butter on top.

Keto zucchini and walnut salad

Made for: Lunch | **Prep Time:** 10 minutes | **Servings:** 1
Per Serving: Kcal: 582, CARBS 7g, PROTEIN 8g, FAT 58g

Ingredients

Dressing
- 1 tbsp olive oil
- 90 ml mayonnaise or vegan mayonnaise
- 1 tsp lemon juice
- ½ garlic clove, finely minced
- ¼ tsp salt
- 1/8 tsp chilli powder

Salad
- ½ (325 g) head of Romaine lettuce
- 55 g (650 ml) arugula lettuce
- 30 ml finely chopped fresh chives or scallions
- 1 (200 g) zucchini

- ½ tbsp olive oil
- salt and pepper
- 120 ml (50 g) chopped walnuts or pecans

Instructions
1. In a small bowl, whisk together all ingredients for the dressing. Reserve the dressing to develop flavor while you make the salad.
2. Trim and cut the salad. Place the Romaine, arugula, and chives in a large bowl.
3. Split the zucchini length-wise and scoop out the seeds. Cut the zucchini halves crosswise into half-inch pieces.
4. Heat olive oil in a frying pan over medium heat until it shimmers. Add zucchini to the pan, and season with salt and pepper. Sauté until lightly browned but still firm.
5. Add the cooked zucchini to the salad, and mix.
6. Roast the nuts briefly in the same pan as the zucchini. Season with salt and pepper. Spoon nuts onto salad, and drizzle with salad dressing.

Keto salmon pie

Made for: Lunch | **Prep Time:** 10 minutes | **Servings:** 1
Per Serving: Kcal: 1025, CARBS 9g, PROTEIN 29g, FAT 96g

Ingredients
Pie crust
- 90 ml (45 g) almond flour
- 30 ml (18 g) sesame seeds
- 30 ml (12 g) coconut flour
- ½ tbsp ground psyllium husk powder
- ½ tsp baking powder
- ½ pinch salt
- 1½ tbsp olive oil or coconut oil
- ½ egg
- 30 ml water

Filling
- 120 ml mayonnaise
- 1½ eggs
- 1 tbsp fresh dill, finely chopped
- ¼ tsp onion powder
- 1/8 tsp ground black pepper
- 70 g (70 ml) of cream cheese at room temperature
- 150 ml (70 g) cheddar cheese, shredded
- 55 g smoked salmon

Instructions
Pie crust
1. Preheat the oven to 350°F (175°C).

2. Place the pie crust ingredients into a food processor bowl fitted with a plastic pastry blade. Pulse until the mixture forms a ball. If you don't have a food processor, you can use a fork to mix the dough.
3. Fit a piece of parchment paper into a 9" (23-cm) springform pan (This makes it a cinch to remove once it's cooked!).
4. Oil your fingers or a spatula, and evenly press the dough into the base and slightly up the sides of the springform pan. Pre-bake the crust for 10–15 minutes, or until lightly browned.

Filling
1. Mix the filling ingredients (except the salmon) in a medium-sized bowl and pour into the pie crust. Add the salmon and bake for 35 minutes or until the pie is golden brown.
2. Let cool for a few minutes and serve with a salad or other vegetables.

Keto quesadillas

Made for: Lunch | **Prep Time:** 10 minutes | **Servings:** 2
Per Serving: Kcal: 487, CARBS 4g, PROTEIN 21g, FAT 42g,

Ingredients
- Low-carb tortillas
- 2 eggs
- 2 egg whites
- 170 g (180 ml) cream cheese
- ½ tsp salt
- 1½ tsp ground psyllium husk powder
- 1 tbsp coconut flour

Filling
- 1 tbsp olive oil or butter for frying
- 140 g (300 ml) Mexican cheese or any hard cheese of your liking
- 28 g (220 ml) baby spinach

Instructions
Tortillas
1. Preheat the oven to 400°F (200°C).
2. Using an electric mixer, beat eggs and egg whites together until fluffy. Add cream cheese and continue to beat until the batter is smooth.
3. In a bowl, combine salt, psyllium husk, and coconut flour. Mix well.
4. Add the flour mixture into the batter while beating. When combined, let the batter sit for a few minutes. It should be thick like pancake batter. Your brand of psyllium husk powder affects this step — be patient... If it does not thicken enough, add some more.

5. Place parchment paper on a baking sheet. Use a spatula to spread the batter over the parchment paper into a big rectangle. You can fry them in a frying pan like pancakes if you want round tortillas.
6. Bake on the upper rack for about 5–10 minutes until the tortilla turns brown around the edges. Keep your eye on the oven — don't let these tasty creations burn on the bottom!
7. Cut the big tortilla into smaller pieces (6 pieces per baking sheet).

Quesadillas
1. Heat oil or butter in a small, non-stick skillet over medium heat.
2. Put a tortilla in the frying pan and sprinkle with cheese, spinach, and some more cheese. Top with another tortilla.
3. Fry each quesadilla for about a minute on each side. You'll know it's done when the cheese melts.

Keto fried halloumi cheese with mushrooms

Made for: Lunch | **Prep Time:** 10 minutes | **Servings:** 2
Per Serving: Kcal: 803, CARBS 7g, PROTEIN 34g, FAT 72g

Ingredients
- 280 g mushrooms
- 280 g halloumi cheese
- 85 g butter
- 10 green olives
- salt and pepper

Instructions
1. Rinse and trim the mushrooms, and cut or slice.
2. Heat a hearty dollop of butter in a frying pan where you can fit both halloumi cheese and mushrooms.
3. Fry the mushrooms on medium heat for 3-5 minutes until golden brown. Season with salt and pepper.
4. If necessary, add more butter and fry the halloumi for a couple of minutes on each side. Stir the mushrooms now and then, and lower the heat towards the end. Serve with olives.

Keto chilli bake

Made for: Lunch | **Prep Time:** 10 minutes | **Servings:** 2
Per Serving: Kcal: 404, CARBS 7g, PROTEIN 30g, FAT 28g

Ingredients
- ½ tbsp olive oil

- 21 g (30 ml) yellow onions, diced
- 1 garlic clove, crushed
- 220 g ground beef
- 21 g (33 ml) red bell peppers, diced
- 21 g (33 ml) green bell peppers, diced
- 1 tsp ground cumin
- ½ tsp chilli powder
- 1 tsp tomato paste
- 110 g (110 ml) crushed tomatoes
- 55 g (120 ml) shredded cheddar cheese
- salt and pepper to taste
- 1 tbsp fresh cilantro, chopped

Instructions
1. Preheat the oven to 350°F (180°C).
2. Dice the onion.
3. Heat a large skillet with olive oil. Add the onion and garlic and fry until soft. Add the ground beef, and cook until all the meat has browned.
4. Add the peppers, stir, and cook until soft.
5. Add the cumin, chilli powder, tomato paste, tomatoes, salt, and pepper, and stir well.
6. Place contents from the pan into a baking dish.
7. Sprinkle the shredded cheese over evenly and cook in the oven for 20 minutes.
8. Garnish with cilantro before serving.

Avocado bacon and chicken bun-less burger

Made for: Lunch | **Prep Time:** 10 minutes | **Servings:** 1
Per Serving: Kcal: 446, CARBS 3g, PROTEIN 41g, FAT 29g

Ingredients
- 750 g ground chicken or ground beef
- 1 (15 g) scallion, finely sliced
- 1 garlic clove, minced
- 1 large egg
- 1 tsp salt
- ½ tsp ground black pepper
- 120 ml (80 g) of red onions, sliced in rings
- 55 g bacon
- 28 g butterhead lettuce, 2 whole leaves per serving
- 1 (200 g) avocado, sliced

Instructions
1. Mix the ground chicken with scallions, garlic, egg, salt, and pepper.
2. Divide the burger mixture into equal portions, one per serving. Shape with your hands into burger patties. Either you make one big per serving or two smaller ones.
3. Fry the onion rings and bacon in a frying pan until the bacon is crispy and the onion has softened. Remove from pan.

4. Add the chicken burgers to the same pan used to fry the onions and the bacon without removing the bacon grease. Fry on both sides until golden and cooked through, 165°F (75°C).
5. Lay one lettuce leaf on a plate. Assemble the burger by placing the bacon, chicken patties, avocado, and cooked onion rings on the lettuce leaf. Fold the lettuce leaf over to become the lettuce "bun."

Quick keto curry bowl

Made for: Lunch | **Prep Time:** 5 minutes | **Servings:** 2
Per Serving: Kcal: 656, CARBS 5g, PROTEIN 47g, FAT 48g

Ingredients
- ½ (55 g) yellow onion, sliced
- ½ tbsp coconut oil
- 1 garlic clove, minced
- 1 tbsp curry powder
- 450 g ground beef or ground turkey
- ¾ tsp salt
- 90 ml coconut cream
- 55 g (425 ml) baby spinach

Instructions
1. steps_item]Peel and slice the onion into half-moons.[/steps_item]
2. Heat a large frying pan or wok with coconut oil. When hot, add the onion and fry until it's soft.
3. Add the garlic and curry powder, stir and cook for another minute. Be careful not to allow the garlic to burn.
4. Add the ground beef, season with salt, and stir until thoroughly cooked.
5. Add the coconut cream and stir to combine.
6. While the curried beef is still simmering in the pan, begin to add the spinach one handful at a time. Stir the spinach with the curried beef until it wilts. Repeat until all the spinach is added. Taste and add more salt if needed.
7. Serve the keto curry in bowls, and enjoy!

Keto pork chops with asparagus

Made for: Lunch | **Prep Time:** 10 minutes | **Servings:** 2
Per Serving: Kcal: 644, CARBS 4g, PROTEIN 48g, FAT47g

Ingredients
- 450 g Pork chops or chicken breasts
- 1/8 tsp salt
- 1/8 tsp pepper

- ½ tbsp Italian seasoning
- ½ tsp onion powder
- 1½ tbsp butter
- 2 garlic cloves, minced
- 60 ml chicken stock or vegetable stock (optional)
- ½ tbsp lemon juice (optional)
- 60 ml heavy whipping cream
- 220 g green asparagus, chopped

Instructions
1. Season your pork chops on both sides with salt, pepper, Italian seasoning, and onion powder.
2. Melt the butter in a skillet on high heat. When the butter is melted, and your pan is hot, add the minced garlic and sauté for a few seconds until fragrant. Add the pork chops and sear for a few minutes on both sides.
3. Pour the broth (if using any), lemon juice, and cream over the seared pork chops. Move the pork chops around a bit to mix the ingredients. Bring to a boil, then reduce the heat to medium.
4. Add the asparagus to the pan. Let the meal simmer for 7-10 minutes, or until the sauce thickens. If the pork chops cook fully before the sauce thickens, remove them and set them to the side while the sauce finishes. Serve and enjoy!

Keto egg casserole with zucchini and ham

Made for: Lunch | **Prep Time:** 10 minutes | **Servings:** 2
Per Serving: Kcal: 363, CARBS 6g, PROTEIN 22g, FAT 28g

Ingredients
- 220 g zucchini, diced (about 0.25 inches or 0.5 centimeters)
- 3 large eggs
- 30 ml whole milk
- 28 g smoked deli ham, diced
- 55 g (55 ml) cream cheese, softened
- ½ (7.5 g) scallion, sliced
- 120 ml (55 g) cheddar cheese, shredded
- salt and pepper, to taste
- ½ tbsp butter for greasing (optional)

Instructions
1. Pre-heat oven to 350° F (180° C). Set aside a lightly greased, 9"x 9" (23 x 23 cm) baking dish.
2. Whisk the eggs and milk together.
3. Add the softened cream cheese. Small lumps of cream cheese in the mix are ok!
4. Add the ham, spring onion, zucchini, and half the amount of shredded cheese. Add salt and pepper to taste.

5. Stir and pour into a greased baking dish. Cover with the remaining shredded cheese.
6. Bake for 20-30 minutes, or until the middle is set.
7. Set aside to cool for 10 minutes before serving.

Keto Thai fish curry and bok choy

Made for: Lunch | **Prep Time:** 10 minutes | **Servings:** 1
Per Serving: Kcal: 658, CARBS 7g, PROTEIN 49g, FAT 48g

Ingredients
- ½ tbsp coconut oil or avocado oil
- 1 tbsp red curry paste
- 180 ml coconut cream
- 120 ml water
- ½ tbsp fish sauce
- 450 g white fish fillets, cubed
- 220 g bok choy, thinly sliced
- salt, to taste

Instructions
1. Heat the oil in a large saucepan, add the curry paste, and fry on moderate heat for 2-3 minutes to activate the spices.
2. Add the coconut cream, water, and fish sauce and bring to a boil.
3. Carefully add the fish pieces and reduce the heat. Simmer for 10 minutes.
4. Add the bok choy and cook for another 3-4 minutes.
5. Serve in large bowls.

Keto salmon-filled avocados

Made for: Lunch | **Prep Time:** 10 minutes | **Servings:** 2
Per Serving: Kcal: 567, CARBS 6g, PROTEIN 26g, FAT 45g

Ingredients
- 2 (400 g) avocados
- 230 g smoked salmon
- 120 ml sour cream
- salt and pepper
- 2 tbsp lemon juice (optional)

Instructions
1. Cut avocados in half and remove the pit.
2. Place a dollop of sour cream, crème Fraiche, or mayonnaise in the hollow of the avocado and add smoked salmon on top.
3. Season to taste with salt and squeeze lemon juice for extra flavor (and keep the avocado from turning brown).

Keto turkey plate

Made for: Lunch | **Prep Time:** 10 minutes | **Servings:** 1
Per Serving: Kcal: 525, CARBS 7g, PROTEIN 26g, FAT 43g

Ingredients
- 230 g deli turkey
- 1 (200 g) avocado, sliced
- 240 ml (35 g) lettuce
- 55 g (55 ml) cream cheese
- 2 tbsp olive oil
- salt and pepper

Instructions
1. Divide the ingredients relevant to the serving number and place an equal amount of turkey, avocado, lettuce, and cream cheese on each plate.
2. Drizzle olive oil over the vegetables and season to taste with salt and pepper.

Keto tuna and avocado salad

Made for: Lunch | **Prep Time:** 10 minutes | **Servings:** 1
Per Serving: Kcal: 639, CARBS 7g, PROTEIN 44g, FAT 45g

Ingredients
- 325 grams of tuna in water
- 1½ (300 g) avocados, cut into eight
- 45 g (70 ml) red bell peppers, sliced
- 28 g (40 ml) red onions, sliced
- 70 g cucumber, quartered
- 28 g (65 ml) celery stalks, diced
- 1 tbsp lime juice
- 40 ml olive oil
- salt and pepper to taste

Instructions
1. Drain the tuna. Use a fork to flake the tuna onto a plate.
2. Slice red bell pepper and red onion into thin slices. Quarter the cucumber lengthways, remove seeds, and slice. Halve the celery lengthways and then cut it into small pieces. Then peel and de-stone the avocado and cut it into eighths.
3. Arrange all ingredients in layers on a large serving platter or individual plates.
4. Place the lime juice and olive oil in a small jar and shake well to combine. Drizzle dressing over salad and finish off with salt and pepper to taste.

Italian plate

Made for: Lunch | **Prep Time:** 10 minutes | **Servings:** 1
Per Serving: Kcal: 561, CARBS 7g, PROTEIN 34g, FAT 43g

Ingredients
- 170 g (350 ml) of fresh mozzarella cheese
- 170 g prosciutto, sliced
- 2 (230 g) tomatoes
- 2 tbsp olive oil
- 10 green olives
- salt and pepper
- fresh basil for garnish

Instructions
1. Put tomatoes, prosciutto, cheese, and olives on a plate. Drizzle with olive oil and season with salt and pepper to taste. Garnish with fresh basil, if desired.

Salad Niçoise

Made for: Lunch | **Prep Time:** 10 minutes | **Servings:** 1
Per Serving: Kcal: 759, CARBS 10g, PROTEIN 52g, FAT 55g

Ingredients

- 2 eggs
- 55 g turnip
- 140 g fresh green beans
- 2 tbsp olive oil
- 1 finely chopped garlic clove (optional)
- 140 g baby gem lettuce or Romaine lettuce
- 55 g cherry tomatoes
- ½ (55 g) red onion
- 350 g tuna in water
- 55 g (100 ml) olives
- salt and pepper

Dressing
2. ½ tbsp Dijon mustard
3. 2 tbsp small capers
4. 14 g anchovies
5. 80 ml water
6. 80 ml mayonnaise
7. 1 tbsp fresh parsley
8. 1 tbsp lemon juice, the juice
9. 1 minced garlic clove (optional)

10. Instructions
11. Mix all the ingredients for the dressing using a mixer or an immersion blender until fully combined and creamy. Set aside.
12. Boil the eggs the way you like them, soft or hard-boiled. Place them immediately in ice-cold water when they are done to make them easier to peel. Cut them into wedges.
13. Wash and peel the turnips. Cut them into 1/2" pieces (1.5cm). Wash and trim the green beans and parboil for 5 minutes in lightly salted water. Use separate pans. Rinse in cold water when done.
14. Place a skillet on medium-high heat and fry the green beans in butter or olive oil. Add finely chopped garlic. Season with salt and pepper.
15. Place lettuce on a serving plate or individual plates. Add tomatoes, onion, drained tuna, eggs, beans, olives, and turnip. Serve with dressing on the side.

Keto tuna salad with boiled eggs

Made for: Lunch | **Prep Time:** 10 minutes | **Servings:** 2
Per Serving: Kcal: 614, CARBS 6g, PROTEIN 33g, FAT 50g

Ingredients
- 110 g (260 ml) celery stalks
- 2 (30 g) scallions
- 140 g tuna in olive oil
- ½ lemon, zest, and juice
- 60 ml mayonnaise
- 1 tsp Dijon mustard
- 4 eggs
- 170 g (850 ml) Romaine lettuce
- 110 g cherry tomatoes
- 2 tbsp olive oil
- salt and pepper

Instructions
1. Chop celery and scallions finely. Add to a medium-sized bowl together with tuna, lemon, mayonnaise, and mustard. Stir to combine, and season with salt and pepper. Set aside.
2. Add eggs to a sauce pan, and add water until it covers the eggs. Bring to a boil and let simmer for 5-6 minutes (soft-medium) or 8-10 minutes (hardboiled).
3. Place in ice-cold water immediately when done to make the eggs easier to peel. Divide them into wedges or halves.
4. Place tuna mix and eggs on a bed of romaine lettuce. Add tomatoes and drizzle olive oil on top. Season with salt and pepper to taste.

Pizza Chicken

Made for: Lunch | **Prep Time:** 10 minutes | **Servings:** 2
Per Serving: Kcal: 380, Carbs (net) 2.5 grams, Protein 41.9 grams, Fat 22.7 grams

Ingredients
- 30ml Olive Oil
- 300g (2 medium) Chicken Breasts
- 100g Tomato Passata plus 50ml water, or 100g Homemade Ketchup
- 1/2 tsp Paprika
- 1/4 tsp Hot Chilli Powder
- 40g Cheddar Cheese, grated (or another cheese of your choice)

Directions
1. Preheat the oven to 180°C.
2. Heat the oil over medium heat in a frying pan.
3. Add the chicken and fry until golden brown on both sides - around 3-4 minutes per side.
4. Remove the chicken from the pan and place it in an ovenproof dish.
5. Return the pan to the heat and add the passata with water, homemade ketchup, paprika, and hot chilli.
6. Cook for 1-2 minutes, and pour the sauce over the chicken.
7. Sprinkle the cheese over the sauce and pop the dish in the oven for 15-20 minutes.

Chicken & Pumpkin Stir Fry

Made for: Lunch | **Prep Time:** 10 minutes | **Servings:** 4
Per Serving: Kcal: 423 Calories / 19.9g Carbs / 37.9g Protein / 20.5g Fat

Ingredients
- 800g Pumpkin - chunky chopped
- 600g Chicken - sliced super thinly
- 100g Leeks - chunky chopped
- 200g Courgette - sliced into strips
- 100g Mushrooms, I'm a particular fan of Chestnut mushrooms, but that's just me! :-) - chunky chopped
- 3 Garlic cloves - chopped finely or 2 tsp garlic puree
- 3 tsp Ginger - chopped finely or 2 tsp ginger puree
- 25g Olive oil
- 25g Butter (for dairy-free, use coconut oil)

- 30g Mixed nuts - roughly chopped (the macros are for mixed nuts, as that was the nuts that I had in). Use any nuts of your choice; just adjust the macros accordingly :-)
- 75g Spinach

The sauce
- 150ml Coconut milk
- 30ml Liquid Aminos (this is a soy sauce replacement)
- 10g Truvia / Natvia / Pure Via Sweetener
- Extra seasoning if needed

Directions
1. Add the olive oil to a large saucepan/wok.
2. Add the leeks & chicken and fry until the chicken is cooked - approx 5-10 minutes.
3. Add the pumpkin, garlic & ginger. Stir through and cook for a further 5 minutes.
4. Now add the mushrooms & courgettes and cook until all the vegetables are cooked through but not mushy. Approx 5 minutes.
5. Finally, add the chopped nuts and spinach, and then add the sauce:
6. The Sauce
7. Add all the sauce ingredients to a bowl, mix and then add to the pan. Gently stir through and cook until the sauce is hot.
8. Enjoy :-)

Keto tuna salad with poached eggs

Made for: Lunch | **Prep Time:** 10 minutes | **Servings:** 2
Per Serving: Kcal: 500, CARBS 5g, PROTEIN 30g, FAT 38g

Ingredients

Tuna salad
- 140 g tuna in water, drained
- 80 ml (35 g) celery stalks, finely chopped
- ½ (55 g) red onion, finely chopped
- 60 ml mayonnaise
- 1 tsp Dijon mustard
- ½ lemon, juice, and zest
- 2 tbsp small capers
- salt and pepper

Poached eggs
- 4 eggs
- 1 tsp salt
- 2 tsp white wine vinegar or white vinegar 5%

Salad
- 55 g cherry tomatoes, halved
- 55 g (230 ml) leafy greens
- 1 tbsp olive oil
- salt, to taste

Instructions

1. Mix all of the ingredients for the tuna salad in a bowl. Set aside.
2. Bring water to a light boil. Add salt and vinegar. Stir the water in circles to create a swirl using a spoon. Crack the egg into the moving water, one at a time.
3. Let the eggs simmer for 3 minutes, and remove them from the water using a slotted spoon.
4. Serve the tuna salad and eggs with your choice of leafy greens and tomatoes. Drizzle with olive oil and season with salt before serving.

Quick Chicken Curry

Made for: Lunch | **Prep Time:** 10 minutes | **Servings:** 4
Per Serving: Kcal: 335, Carbs (net) 7.8 grams, Protein 31.1 grams, Fat 19.1 grams

Ingredients

- 600g Chicken Breast, diced into approx 2cm chunks
- 100g Leeks, thinly sliced
- 150g Red Pepper (approx. 1 medium), diced
- 150g Green Pepper (approx. 1 medium), diced
- 400g Tinned Chopped Tomatoes
- 400g Tinned Coconut Milk
- 5 tsp Curry Blend (or other good quality curry powder)
- 1/2 tsp Kashmiri Chilli
- 1/2 tsp Garlic Powder (optional)
- Seasoning
- Handful Spinach (optional)
- 1 tbsp Olive Oil for frying

Directions

1. Pop the olive oil in the pan and saute the leeks until soft (about 2-3 minutes).
2. Now add the peppers and fry for a further 5 minutes.
3. Add all the spices and chicken and stir well. Fry for a couple more minutes.
4. Add to this coconut milk and tinned tomatoes.
5. Stir well, bring to boil, and turn down to a simmer.
6. Simmer for about 30 minutes.
7. Season to taste.

Roast Chicken Thighs with Lemon

Made for: Lunch | **Prep Time:** 20 minutes | **Servings:** 4
Per Serving: Kcal: 426, 2.6g Carbs, 46.5g Protein, 25.5g Fat

Ingredients

- 1 kg (6-8) Chicken Thighs
- 1 Wax-free Lemon
- 2-3 Garlic Cloves, finely sliced
- 15ml Olive Oil
- Pink Himalayan / Rock / Sea Salt & Black Pepper
- 300g Asparagus Tips
- Optional: 100ml Chicken Stock
- 30ml (30g) Double Cream
- Optional: 1/2 tsp Arrowroot Powder

Directions

1. Cut slits into each chicken thigh and place in a large bowl.
2. Slice the lemon into thin slices and add to the bowl.
3. Add the garlic, olive oil, salt, and pepper. Massage into the chicken.
4. Leave to rest for 30 minutes or place in a food bag and store in the fridge overnight.
5. Lay the chicken thighs in a roasting tray and spread the lemon slices in and around each thigh.
6. Roast uncovered for 30 minutes at 200°C.
7. Add the asparagus on top of the chicken thighs and baste everything with the juices from the thighs. If your dish needs extra fluid, add the chicken stock or a little water. There should be plenty of flavour in the tray from the chicken :)
8. Return to the oven and roast for 15-20 mins until golden.
9. Once cooked, place the chicken and asparagus in a serving dish.
10. To make a creamy gravy, transfer the liquid to a small sauce pan over high heat, bring to boil, and add the double cream. Quickly whisk together and serve.
11. Mix 1/2 tsp arrowroot powder in a little cold water for a thicker sauce and add to the sauce, whisking.

Ross's Chicken Doner Kebab

Made for: Lunch | **Prep Time:** 15 minutes | **Servings:** 6
Per Serving: Kcal: 373, 2.7g Carbs, 32.6g Protein, 26g Fat

Ingredients

- 1kg Chicken Thighs, boneless and skinless
- 150g Greek or Greek Style Yogurt
- 1 tbsp Paprika
- 1 tbsp Ground Cumin
- 1/4 tsp Cayenne Pepper or Kashmiri Chilli
- 4 Garlic Cloves
- Juice of 1 Lemon
- 3 tbsp (45ml) Olive Oil

- 1/2 tsp Freshly Ground Black Pepper
- 50g Shallot
- 3 tsp Oregano
- Optional: 1 swede, peeled and chopped in half to use as a base

Directions
1. Blitz the shallot and garlic cloves in a small food processor or a Nutri-bullet blender.
2. Mix all ingredients in a bowl and marinade overnight in the fridge - the longer, the better.
3. Take a big chunk out of a swede (e.g., chop it in half) to use as the base. Stick the skewers into the swede to point straight up (if using wooden skewers, soak in water for 30 minutes first).
4. Stack the chicken thighs onto the skewers, alternating the directions of the thighs. Pour any leftover marinade on top.
5. Cook for 1 hr 45 minutes at 180°C, or anywhere between 1 hour & 30 minutes to 2 hours.
6. Once cooked, either shave pieces off using a knife (as shown in the photo) or cut it all up and pan fry the pieces when you want them!

Sandie's Golden Kebabs

Made for: Lunch | **Prep Time:** 20 minutes | **Servings:** 4
Per Serving: Kcal: 292, Carbs (net) 6.6 grams, Protein 37 grams, Fat 12.7 grams

Ingredients
- 300g Chicken Mini Fillets
- 100g Courgette, cut into 1 cm slices
- 100g Aubergine, cut into 1 cm slices
- 100g Button Mushrooms
- 100g Green Pepper, sliced into small chunks
- 20ml Olive Oil
- 1/2 tsp Ground Turmeric
- 2 Garlic Cloves / 5g Garlic Puree
- 1/2 inch Fresh Ginger / 5g Ginger Puree

Directions
1. If you're not a fan of one of the veggies, there are plenty of alternatives - Broccoli / Cauli Florets, Asparagus, or even a few baby plum tomatoes.
2. Create your kebabs on wooden or metal skewers and set them on a tray ready for the marinade.

3. Use a small food processor / Nutri-bullet blender or a pestle and mortar to create a paste with the oil, turmeric, garlic, and ginger
4. Spoon the paste over the kebabs. Hold some back for part way through the cooking process.
5. Cooking Options
6. These work great in our Air Fryer, which took about 15 minutes at 200°C.
7. You can oven bake these at 200°C for about 25-30 minutes. Check that the chicken is fully cooked.
8. Or fry in a griddle pan over medium heat for around 10-15 minutes and get that authentic BBQ scoring.
9. Part way through the cooking process, spoon over the remainder of the paste.

Shrimp salad with hot bacon fat dressing

Made for: Lunch | **Prep Time:** 5 minutes | **Servings:** 2
Per Serving: Kcal: 495, CARBS 3g, PROTEIN 24g, FAT 42g

Ingredients
Spinach salad
- 1 tbsp ghee or butter
- 220 g medium shrimp, raw, peeled, and deveined
- 1 garlic clove, coarsely chopped
- 85 g (650 ml) of fresh baby spinach
- 1 hard-boiled egg, chopped
- 28 g bacon, cooked and chopped
- 14 g parmesan cheese, finely grated (optional)
- salt and pepper, to taste

Hot bacon fat dressing
- 60 ml bacon fat or light olive oil
- 30 ml apple cider vinegar
- ½ tbsp Dijon mustard
- salt
- ground black pepper

Instructions
1. In a large pan over medium-high heat, melt butter.
2. Pat the shrimp dry with a paper towel to remove as much moisture as possible. Add the shrimp and the garlic to the skillet and sauté for 3-5 minutes until the shrimp are bright pink and thoroughly cooked. Remove shrimp from the heat.
3. Equally distribute the spinach among the plates, followed by the hard-boiled eggs, bacon, shrimp, and parmesan cheese.

4. In a small saucepan, over medium heat, melt the bacon fat. Add the apple cider vinegar and remaining ingredients, whisking until well combined.
5. Dress salad plates with hot bacon vinaigrette and serve immediately.

Smothered Chicken

Made for: Lunch | **Prep Time:** 15 minutes | **Servings:** 4
Per Serving: Kcal: 439, 1.8g Carbs, 47g Protein, 26.8g Fat

Ingredients
- 4 Chicken Breasts (150-200g each)
- 15g Butter
- 8 Rashers (around 160g) of Streaky Bacon
- 100g Shallots
- 100g Mushrooms or Bell Pepper
- 100g Mascarpone (this can be replaced with Soft Cream Cheese)
- A handful of fresh parsley, finely chopped
- Salt & Pepper

Directions
1. Flatten or butterfly the chicken breasts and grill for around 10-15 minutes until fully cooked. Alternatively, start the chicken breasts off in a pan and transfer them to the oven to finish cooking.
2. Heat the butter in a medium sauce pan over gentle heat.
3. Chop the bacon and shallots - add these to the pan and allow to cook gently.
4. Chop the mushrooms/peppers and after a few minutes, add them to the pan along with the bacon & shallots.
5. Once the bacon is cooked and the shallots & peppers have softened, add the mascarpone to the pan and let it melt into a sauce.
6. If your mascarpone is quite thick, add a dash of milk (of your choice) to the sauce and stir in.
7. Add the parsley (save some for serving) to the sauce and allow it to cook through until it reaches your preferred consistency.
8. Once the chicken breasts are cooked, transfer them to a dish, season the sauce to taste, and pour them on top.

Spanish Chicken

Made for: Lunch | **Prep Time:** 15 minutes | **Servings:** 4
Per Serving: Kcal: 408, Carbs (net) 5.6 grams, Protein 32.7 grams, Fat 28.2 grams

Ingredients
- 600g Skinned Chicken Thigh Fillets
- 40g Butter or 40ml Olive Oil
- 100g Leeks, finely sliced
- 80g Red Pepper, diced
- 2 Garlic Cloves, finely chopped
- 200g (half a tin) Chopped Tomatoes
- 60g Diced / Sliced Chorizo
- 1-2 tsp Smoked Paprika
- 1 tsp Dried Thyme
- 200ml Chicken Stock or 1 Stock Cube

Directions
1. Arrange the chicken thighs in the slow cooker.
2. Heat the oil/butter over medium heat in a medium frying pan. When it's hot, add the leek, pepper, and garlic. Fry gently for 5 minutes for them to soften a little and start to turn golden. Remove from the heat.
3. Add the chopped tomatoes to the chicken.
4. Add the leeks, pepper, garlic, and chorizo.
5. Sprinkle the paprika and thyme over the dish.
6. Pour in the chicken stock and set the slow cooker to low to allow it to cook all day (around 8 hours). It'll take around 4 hours on a high setting.
7. Before serving, add a little soured cream or, for a thicker sauce, mix a teaspoon of arrowroot powder with 20ml cold water and stir into the sauce. Allow thickening for 5 minutes.

Without a slow cooker:
1. To make this dish without a slow cooker, it's better to use chicken breast (quickly pan fry this before adding to an ovenproof dish). Follow the other steps as normal, placing everything in the dish rather than the slow cooker, and bake for around 35-40 minutes at 180°C.

Spicy Chicken Skewers

Made for: Lunch | **Prep Time:** 5 minutes | **Servings:** 8
Per Serving: Kcal: 128, Carbs (net) 1.2 grams, Protein 24.7 grams, Fat 2.7 grams

Ingredients
- 800g Diced Chicken Breast
- 120g Greek or Greek-Style Yogurt
- Salt and Pepper
- 3 tsp Curry Blend
- 1/2 tsp Garlic Powder
- 1/2 tsp Kashmiri Chilli
- Kebab Sticks, cut in half

Directions

2. Add all the spices and seasoning to the yogurt and mix
3. Add the chicken and mix. Leave to marinate for 30 minutes, preferably 1 hour
4. Roughly 4 chunks of chicken per kebab stick
5. Bake at 180C for 20 - 25minutes

Sweet & Sour Chicken

Made for: Lunch | **Prep Time:** 15 minutes | **Servings:** 4
Per Serving: Kcal: 714, 9.3g Carbs, 71.2g Protein, 42.5g Fat

Ingredients
- 500g Chicken Breast
- 140ml Water
- 100g Pork Scratchings (Shop bought or made your own using this recipe here)
- 70g Ketchup - Can be the Ketoroma one or Liam's Sauce
- 65g Truvia / Nat Via / Pure Via Sweetener
- 1 Egg
- 50g Grated Parmesan Cheese
- 50g Apple Cider Vinegar
- 50g Sesame Oil
- 50g Shallots
- 50g Green Pepper
- 40g Lupin Flour
- 2 Tbsp Coconut Aminos (Soy Sauce Alternative)
- 2 tsp Chilli Powder
- 1.5 tsp Garlic Powder
- 0.5 tsp Salt
- 1 tsp Onion Powder
- 1.5tsp Xantham Gum
- 0.5tsp Black Pepper

Directions
The Chicken

2. Heat the Oven / Air Fryer to 200°C and line a try with baking parchment.
3. Put the pork scratchings into a food processor and blitz into a fine crumb. Pour the Parmesan, lupin, chili powder, garlic powder, onion powder, sea salt, and pepper into a medium-sized bowl. Mix well and then set aside.
4. Whisk the egg with 60ml water until fully combined in a shallow bowl. Chop the chicken breasts into 1- 1.5" pieces and set them aside.

5. Dip a piece of chicken in the egg wash with one hand and then place it into the breading bowl without touching the pork rinds. On the other hand, toss the chicken around in the pork rinds and put it on the baking sheet. Repeat for all the chicken pieces and spread them evenly around the baking sheet. Double dip the chicken in the egg wash and again in the breading until all the pork rinds have been used up.
6. Bake in the preheated oven for 18-20 minutes until the chicken is golden. While the chicken is in the oven, make the sauce.

The Sauce
1. Chop up an onion and a dash of green pepper and heat a pan on medium-high heat with half of the sesame oil. Fry the pepper and onion until they have softened and brown.
2. In a medium-sized mixing bowl, whisk xanthan gum with the rest of the sesame oil. Pour in the apple cider vinegar, ketchup, water, sweetener, and soy sauce, and whisk well to combine. Pour into the hot pan with the pepper and onion and bring up to a simmer. Cook until thick, 1-2 minutes, then carefully mix the baked chicken.
3. Serve hot over Cauliflower Fried Rice

Tandoori Chicken

Made for: Lunch | **Prep Time:** 15 minutes | **Servings:** 6
Per Serving: Kcal: 220, Carbs (net) 3.4 grams, Protein 23.2 grams, Fat 12.9 grams

Ingredients
Part 1

- 6 Chicken Thighs, skinless
- Juice of 1/2 a Lemon
- 1 tsp Kashmiri Chilli

Part 2

- A whole bulb of Garlic (approx. 10-12 cloves), crushed
- 4 inches Ginger, crushed
- 3 tbsp (45g Greek or Greek Style Yogurt (for dairy-free, replace this with Coconut Yogurt)
- 1 level tbsp Pink Himalayan / Rock / Sea Salt
- 1 tbsp Kashmiri Chilli
- 1 tbsp Garam Masala
- 10g Fresh Coriander finely chopped

Directions
Part 1

1. Wash the chicken thoroughly and then cut slices into the flesh to allow the marinade to work its magic.
2. Squeeze the lemon juice, sprinkle the Kashmiri chilli on the chicken, and massage it into the meat. Leave in the fridge for an hour.

Part 2

1. Add all the ingredients into a bowl with the chicken, mix thoroughly, and leave in the fridge overnight.
2. Take this out of the fridge at least an hour or two before you cook.
3. Separate the pieces if you are going to cook in the oven or grill - otherwise, it'll turn into a stew.
4. Cook for around 25 minutes on high heat, turning regularly to ensure it doesn't burn, but you want it to take on some charred flavour. If you are cooking on a BBQ, the same principles apply.
5. Serve with wedges of lemons & limes and chopped coriander.

Teesside Hotshot Parmo

Made for: Lunch | **Prep Time:** 15 minutes | **Servings:** 2
Per Serving: Kcal: 693, Carbs (net) 5.3 grams, Protein 68.7 grams, Fat 43.1 grams

Ingredients

- 1 x 90-second bread roll, toasted well and blitzed into crumbs, transferred to a large dish
- 2 Chicken Breasts (360g)
- 1 Egg, whisked, in a large dish
- 15g Coconut Flour in a large dish
- 30g Mascarpone
- 50ml Soured Cream
- 40g Grated Mozzarella
- 40g Mature Grated Cheddar
- 1 tsp Jalapenos, chopped finely
- 15g Pepperoni
- 15g Butter/ Olive oil

Directions

1. Preheat the oven to 180°C.
2. Prepare your 90-second bread as per the recipe. Slice in half and toast.
3. Use a meat hammer or large rolling pin to flatten your chicken breasts and season well
4. Line up your 3 large dishes......
5. Coconut flour
6. Whisked eggs
7. Put your toasted bread in the food processor and blitz until a fine crumb. Place into a large dish

8. Dip each chicken breast on both sides into the coconut powder, then the whisked egg, and coat well before placing it into your bowl of breadcrumbs and coat well
9. In a frying pan, melt your butter and lightly fry the chicken on both sides for about 30 seconds. It'll be nice and golden
10. Now put onto a baking tray and pop in the oven for about 12 minutes or until completely cooked
11. Place your mascarpone, mozzarella, and sour cream into a small pan on low and melt until a smooth sauce is formed; keep stirring till this happens
12. Remove the cooked chicken from the oven.
13. Pour the sauce evenly over each piece of chicken
14. Then sprinkle the cheddar over the chicken
15. Finally, sprinkle with the chopped pepperoni and Jalapenos
16. Place back in the oven until the cheese has melted and is bubbling

Thai Green Curry Paste & Chicken Curry

Made for: Lunch | **Prep Time:** 15 minutes | **Servings:** 2
Per Serving: Kcal: 573, 6g Carbs, 51g Protein, 39g Fat

Ingredients
Thai Green Curry Paste

- 4-6 Medium Green Chillies, de-seeded and roughly chopped
- 100g Shallots or Spring Onions, roughly chopped
- 20g Fresh Ginger, peeled and roughly chopped
- 2 Garlic Cloves, peeled
- Small bunch of Fresh Coriander (stalks included)
- 2 Lemongrass Stalks, chopped (or 2 tbsp dried)
- Juice & Zest of 1 Lime
- 8 Kaffir Lime Leaves, torn into pieces (or add the zest of a second lime)
- 1 tbsp Coriander Seeds, crushed
- 1 tsp Ground Cumin
- 1 tsp Ground Turmeric
- 1 tsp Black Peppercorns, crushed
- 2 tsp Coconut Aminos (or a light Soy Sauce)
- 45g Coconut Oil, melted

Thai Green Chicken Curry

- 300-400g Chicken Breast, diced

- 200g Coconut Milk (as high % coconut extract as you can get - we used Lidl's 91%)
- 20g Coconut Oil
- 2 portions of Thai Curry Paste (see above)

Directions
Thai Green Curry Paste
1. Add all of the paste ingredients to a small food processor and blitz in 15-20 second bursts until you've created a paste.
2. Store in the fridge for around 10-14 days or freeze in individual portions (e.g., in an ice cube tray), ready to make a quick curry :)

Thai Green Chicken Curry
1. Heat the oil in a medium saucepan/wok.
2. Fry the diced chicken over medium heat for 3 - 5 minutes, ensuring the chicken has been sealed on all sides.
3. Add the curry paste and cook over medium heat for 2 - 3 minutes.
4. Add the coconut milk and thoroughly mix with the chicken and paste.
5. Bring to boil and then reduce to a simmer for another 3 - 5 minutes.
6. Check one of the larger chicken pieces to ensure it is cooked through.

Keto Italian cabbage stir-fry

This meal is simple rustic deliciousness. The combination of tart cabbage, luscious basil, and savory beef is melt-in-your-mouth fabulous. This is keto at its finest.

Made for: Lunch | **Prep Time:** 10 minutes | **Servings:** 2
Per Serving: Kcal: 966, CARBS 9g, PROTEIN 32g, FAT 88g

Ingredients
- 325 g green cabbage
- 70 g butter, divided
- 280 g ground beef
- ½ tbsp white wine vinegar
- ½ tsp salt
- ½ tsp onion powder
- 1/8 tsp pepper
- 1 tbsp tomato paste
- 1 garlic clove, finely chopped
- 45 g leeks, thinly sliced
- 9 g (50 ml) fresh basil, chopped
- 120 ml mayonnaise or sour cream for serving

Instructions
1. Shred the green cabbage finely with a sharp knife or food processor.
2. In a large frying pan, melt half of the butter over medium heat. Add the cabbage and fry for about 10 minutes, or until just softened.
3. Add vinegar, salt, onion powder, and pepper. Stir and fry for 2-3 minutes, or until well incorporated. Transfer the sauteed cabbage to a large bowl.
4. Heat the rest of the butter in the pan. Add the garlic and leeks, and sauté for a minute.
5. Add meat, and continue frying until cooked through. Sauté until most of the liquid has evaporated.
6. Add tomato paste and mix well. Lower the heat a little and add reserved cabbage and fresh basil. Stir until cooked through.
7. Adjust seasoning and serve with a dollop of sour cream or mayonnaise.

Keto chili bake

Made for: Lunch | **Prep Time:** 10 minutes | **Servings:** 2
Per Serving: Kcal: 404, CARBS 7g, PROTEIN 30g, FAT 28g

Ingredients
- 1 tbsp olive oil
- 45 g (65 ml) yellow onions, diced
- 2 garlic cloves, crushed
- 450 g ground beef
- 45 g (70 ml) red bell peppers, diced
- 45 g (70 ml) green bell peppers, diced
- 2 tsp ground cumin
- 1 tsp chili powder
- 2 tsp tomato paste
- 230 g (220 ml) crushed tomatoes
- 110 g (230 ml) shredded cheddar cheese
- salt and pepper to taste
- 2 tbsp fresh cilantro, chopped

Instructions
1. Preheat the oven to 350°F (180°C).
2. Dice the onion.
3. Heat up a large skillet with olive oil. Add the onion and garlic and fry until soft. Add the ground beef, and cook until all the meat has browned.
4. Add the peppers, stir, and cook until soft.
5. Add the cumin, chili powder, tomato paste, tomatoes, salt, and pepper, and stir well.
6. Place contents from the pan into a baking dish.
7. Sprinkle the shredded cheese over evenly and cook in the oven for 20 minutes.
8. Garnish with cilantro before serving.

DINNER RECIPE

Seafood salad with avocado

A fresh and tasty seafood salad with shrimp and salmon is an excellent source of protein. When added to avocado, mayonnaise, and sour cream, healthy fats make this a superb keto meal. If you're dairy-free, omit the sour cream and add more mayo.

Made for: Dinner | **Prep Time:** 10 minutes | **Servings:** 1
Per Serving: Kcal: 444, CARBS 3g, PROTEIN 35g, FAT 32g

Ingredients
- Salad dressing
- 1/3 tbsp lime juice
- 20 ml mayonnaise
- 13 ml sour cream
- 1/6 garlic clove, minced
- 1/6 tsp salt
- 10 ml (7 g) red onions, finely minced
- 7 ml white pepper

Seafood salad
- 75 g shrimp, cooked, chopped
- 75 g cooked salmon, boneless fillets, bite-sized pieces
- 12 g (16 ml) tomatoes, chopped (optional)
- 7 g cucumber, deseeded, finely chopped
- 1/6 (35 g) avocado, chopped
- 1/3 tbsp fresh basil, roughly sliced

Instructions
1. Combine lime juice, mayonnaise, sour cream, garlic, salt, pepper, and onion in a mixing bowl. Set aside.
2. Toss together salmon, shrimp, avocado, cucumber, and tomato in a larger bowl.
3. Pour mayonnaise dressing over the seafood and vegetables and toss gently to combine.
4. Let chill 20-30 minutes before serving.

Keto oven-baked Brie cheese

Elegant. Creamy. Comforting. Keto. Enjoy the exquisite flavor of warm Brie, paired with a savory blend of fresh herbs and toasted nuts. Your next cocktail party just got easier! Brie works beautifully as a dessert course, too.

Made for: Dinner | **Prep Time:** 5 minutes | **Servings:** 1
Per Serving: Kcal: 341, CARBS 1g, PROTEIN 15g, FAT 31g

Ingredients
- 65 g Brie cheese or Camembert cheese
- ¼ garlic clove, minced
- ¼ tbsp fresh rosemary, coarsely chopped
- 14 g pecans or walnuts, coarsely chopped
- ¼ tbsp olive oil
- salt and pepper

Instructions
1. Instructions are for 4 servings. Please modify as needed.
2. Preheat the oven to 400°F (200°C).
3. Place the cheese on a sheet pan lined with parchment paper or a small nonstick baking dish.
4. Mix the garlic, herb, and nuts with olive oil in a small bowl. Add salt and pepper to taste.
5. Place the nut mixture on the cheese and bake for 10 minutes or until the cheese is warm and soft and the nuts are toasted. Serve warm or lukewarm.

Keto lasagna

Made for: Dinner | **Prep Time:** 10 minutes | **Servings:** 2
Per Serving: Kcal: 752, CARBS 8g, PROTEIN 41g, FAT 60g

Ingredients

Lasagna sheets
- 22/3 eggs, beaten
- 95 g (100 ml) cream cheese
- 1/3 tsp salt
- 25 ml (16 g) ground psyllium husk powder

Meat sauce
- 1 tbsp olive oil
- 1/6 (18 g) yellow onion, finely chopped
- 1/3 garlic clove, finely chopped
- 220 g ground beef or ground turkey
- 2/3 tbsp tomato paste
- 1/6 tbsp dried basil
- 1/3 tsp salt
- 1/10 tsp ground black pepper
- 40 ml water

Cheese topping
- 120 ml sour cream
- 80 ml (38 g) shredded mozzarella cheese
- 40 ml (13 g) shredded Parmesan cheese
- 1/6 tsp salt
- 1/10 tsp ground black pepper
- 40 ml (2.7 g) fresh parsley, finely chopped

Instructions

Lasagna sheets
1. Preheat the oven to 300°F (150°C). Line a baking sheet with parchment paper.
2. In a medium-sized bowl, whisk together the ingredients until a smooth batter. Gradually whisk in the psyllium husk, and then set aside for a few minutes.

3. Add the batter to the center of the parchment paper, and then place another parchment paper on top. Flatten with a rolling pin until the batter is at least 13 x 18" (33 x 45 cm). If you prefer thinner pasta, you can divide the batter into two equal batches, placing it on two baking sheets with parchment paper.
4. Bake each sheet (with parchment paper) for about 10-12 minutes. Set aside to cool. Next, remove the paper and slice pasta into sheets that fit a 9 x 12" (23 x 30 cm) baking dish.

Meat sauce
1. In a large pan, over medium-high heat, warm the olive oil. Add the onion and garlic, stirring until soft. Next, add the beef, tomato paste, and spices, and combine thoroughly until the beef is no longer pink.
2. Add water to the mixture, bring to a boil, lower the heat, and let simmer for at least 15 minutes or until most of the water has evaporated. The sauce should be drier since these lasagna sheets don't soak up as much liquid as traditional ones. Set aside.
3. Preheat the oven to 400°F (200°C). Grease a 9 x 12" (23 x 30 cm) baking dish.

Cheese topping
1. Mix the mozzarella cheese with sour cream and most of the parmesan cheese. Reserve two tablespoons of parmesan cheese for the final topping. Add salt and pepper and stir in the parsley.
2. Alternately layer the pasta sheets and meat sauce in the baking dish, starting with the pasta, followed by the meat sauce.
3. Spread the cheese mixture on the pasta, and finish with the extra parmesan cheese.
4. Bake in the oven for about 30 minutes or until the lasagna has a nicely browned surface. Serve with a green salad and your favorite dressing.

Keto pizza

Made for: Dinner | **Prep Time:** 10 minutes | **Servings:** 2
Per Serving: Kcal: 1024, CARBS 6g, PROTEIN 56g, FAT 86g

Ingredients

Crust
- 4 eggs
- 350 ml (170 g) shredded mozzarella cheese

Topping
- 3 tbsp unsweetened tomato sauce
- 1 tsp dried oregano
- 300 ml (170 g) shredded provolone cheese
- 45 g pepperoni
- olives (optional)

For serving
- 55 g (230 ml) leafy greens
- 60 ml olive oil
- salt and ground black pepper

Instructions
1. Preheat the oven to 400°F (200°C).
2. Start by making the crust. Crack eggs into a medium-sized bowl and add shredded cheese. Give it a good stir to combine.
3. Use a spatula to spread the cheese and egg batter on a baking sheet lined with parchment paper. You can form two circles or just make one large rectangular pizza. Bake in the oven for 15 minutes until the pizza crust turns golden. Remove and let cool for a minute or two.
4. Increase the oven temperature to 450°F (225°C).
5. Spread tomato sauce on the crust and sprinkle oregano on top. Top with cheese, and place the pepperoni and olives on top.
6. Bake for another 5-10 minutes or until the pizza has turned a golden brown color.
7. Serve with a fresh salad on the side.

Low-carb curry chicken zucchini boats

Made for: Dinner | **Prep Time:** 10 minutes | **Servings:** 2
Per Serving: Kcal: 636, CARBS 8g, PROTEIN 47g, FAT 45g

Ingredients
- 450 g zucchini
- ½ tsp salt
- 220 g chicken breasts, chopped into small pieces
- ½ tbsp olive oil
- ½ tbsp butter
- 1 tbsp mayonnaise
- 70 g (80 ml) cottage cheese
- ½ tbsp yellow curry powder
- ½ tsp onion powder
- 240 ml (110 g) gouda cheese, shredded
- salt and pepper

For serving
- ¼ tbsp red wine vinegar
- salt and pepper
- 2 tbsp olive oil
- 85 g (550 ml) lettuce

Instructions

1. Preheat the oven to 375°F (190°C). Grease a 9 x 12" (22 x 30 cm) baking dish.
2. Split each zucchini in half, lengthwise, and remove the seeds with a spoon. Sprinkle with salt and let sit for 10 minutes.
3. Blot off the drops of liquid with paper towels. Place the halves in a greased baking dish.
4. Warm the olive oil and butter over medium-high heat in a large pan. Add the chicken, season with salt and pepper, and saute until done. Transfer to a medium-sized bowl to cool.
5. Mix the chicken, mayonnaise, cottage cheese, spices, and a third of the grated cheese. Season to taste.
6. Distribute the mixture into the zucchini halves and sprinkle the remaining cheese on top. Bake for approximately 35-40 minutes or until the zucchini boats have turned a nice golden color.
7. Mix oil, vinegar, salt, and pepper into a simple vinaigrette. Serve the zucchini boats beside a simple salad made with lettuce and vinaigrette.

Classic keto steak tartare

Made for: Dinner | **Prep Time:** 10 minutes | **Servings:** 2
Per Serving: Kcal: 357, CARBS 6g, PROTEIN 42g, FAT 17g

Ingredients
- 280 g beef, tenderloin
- ½ (55 g) yellow onion
- 2 tbsp small capers
- 2 tbsp Dijon mustard
- 2 tbsp parmesan cheese
- 1 tbsp fresh horseradish, grated
- 2 eggs
- 45 g baby gem lettuce
- 55 g canned beets, diced
- 1 tbsp fresh parsley, finely chopped
- coarse salt
- ground black pepper

Instructions
1. Finely chop the onion, beets, and parsley.
2. Shred the parmesan and horseradish.
3. Rinse the salad and place them on the plate.
4. Finely chop or grind the beef (your local butcher can also provide this service for you). Divide into equal parts, one per serving. Shape into patties with an indentation in the center.

5. Separate the eggs, and set aside each yolk in one half of an egg shell. The egg white will not be used for this recipe but save it in the fridge in an air-tight container for other recipes or omelets.
6. Serve each patty on a plate. Spread the onion, beets, capers, parmesan, and small dollops of Dijon mustard around the patty. Sprinkle horseradish and parsley on top.
7. Finally, position the egg yolk in the center of each patty. Serve with salt and pepper to taste.

Keto harvest pumpkin and sausage soup

Made for: Dinner | **Prep Time:** 10 minutes | **Servings:** 2
Per Serving: Kcal: 522, CARBS 5g PROTEIN 33g, FAT 41g

Ingredients
- 325 g fresh sausage
- 7 g white onions, minced
- ½ (60 g) small red bell pepper, diced
- ½ garlic clove, minced
- ½ pinch salt
- ¼ tsp rubbed dried sage
- ¼ tsp ground dried thyme
- ¼ tsp red chili peppers flakes (optional)
- 60 ml pumpkin puree or crushed tomatoes
- 180 ml chicken broth
- 60 ml heavy whipping cream
- Heavy whipping cream
- Also known as thickened cream or double cream
- ½ tbsp salted butter

Instructions
1. Use a large skillet to brown the sausage, onion, and pepper on medium-high heat.
2. When pork is thoroughly cooked, and the onions and pepper are browned (about 10 to 15 minutes), sprinkle in the seasonings and stir to mix.
3. Stir in the pumpkin, broth, and cream. Simmer uncovered on low heat for 15 to 20 minutes or until the soup has thickened.
4. Add the butter, stir well, and serve warm.

Keto tortilla pizza

Made for: Dinner | **Prep Time:** 10 minutes | **Servings:** 2
Per Serving: Kcal: 378, CARBS 6g PROTEIN 21g FAT 30g

Ingredients

Low-carb tortillas
- 1 large egg

- 1 large, egg white
- 85 g (90 ml) of cream cheese at room temperature
- 1/8 tsp salt
- ½ tsp ground psyllium husk powder
- ½ tbsp coconut flour

Topping
- 60 ml unsweetened tomato sauce, divided
- 240 ml (110 g) shredded mozzarella cheese
- 1 tsp dried basil or dried oregano

Instructions

Tortillas
1. Preheat the oven to 400°F (200°C). Set aside (2) baking sheets lined with parchment paper.
2. Add the eggs and egg whites to a large mixing bowl. Using an electric mixer, whisk together for a few minutes until fluffy. Add the cream cheese, and whisk together until it becomes a smooth batter.
3. Mix the salt, psyllium husk, and coconut flour in a small bowl. Add one spoonful of this mixture into the batter, whisk together, and repeat until combined. Let the batter sit for a few minutes or until the batter has thickened (see tip).
4. Use a spatula to spread the batter on the baking sheets into 4-6 thin circles or 2 thin rectangles (no more than ¼" or 5 mm thick).
5. Bake on the middle and upper racks for about 15 minutes or until lightly browned the edges are. Remove from oven, and set aside.

Pizza
1. Increase the oven temperature to 450°F (225°C).
2. Spread the tomato sauce onto each crust, top with the cheese, basil, or oregano, and return to middle and upper oven racks.
3. Bake for about 5 minutes, or until the cheese is melted and golden. Set aside to cool for a few minutes, then slice, and serve.

Steak with keto mushroom sauce

Made for: Dinner | **Prep Time:** 10 minutes | **Servings:** 2
Per Serving: Kcal: 650, CARBS 7g, PROTEIN 48g, FAT 48g

Ingredients

Steak

- 450 g ribeye steaks, 1 steak per serving
- ½ tbsp ghee or butter
- salt and ground black pepper to taste

Mushroom sauce
- ½ tbsp butter
- 1 garlic clove, crushed
- 60 ml mushrooms, sliced
- 40 ml (40 g) cream cheese
- 60 ml heavy whipping cream
- salt and ground black pepper to taste

Salad
- 240 ml (55 g) leafy greens
- ½ (55 g) tomato, diced

Instructions

Steak
1. Take your steaks out of the fridge and bring them to room temperature.
2. Dry the steaks with a paper towel and season generously with salt and pepper.
3. Heat a large frying pan on medium to high heat, depending on how you like your steak cooked. Add the butter (or preferably the ghee as it had a higher smoke point). Place the steaks in the frying pan and fry to your liking: rare, medium, or well done. Remove the meat from the pan, cover, and let it rest while preparing the rest.

Mushroom sauce
1. Lower the heat and add more butter (if necessary) to the same frying pan. Fry the garlic and mushroom slices until golden. Season with salt and pepper.
2. Turn the heat down and mix the cream cheese to avoid lumps.
3. Add the cream and stir until heated through. Taste and season with more salt and pepper if necessary.

Serving
1. Serve the steaks with creamy mushroom sauce and salad.

Keto roast beef and cheddar plate

Made for: Dinner | **Prep Time:** 10 minutes | **Servings:** 2
Per Serving: Kcal: 838, CARBS 6g, PROTEIN 40g, FAT 70g

Ingredients
- 230 g deli roast beef, rolled
- 140 g (290 ml) cheddar cheese, cut into finger-like slices
- 1 (200 g) avocado, sliced
- 6 radishes, sliced
- 1 (15 g) scallion, cut at an angle
- 4 tbsp mayonnaise
- 1 tbsp Dijon mustard

- 55 g (350 ml) lettuce
- 1 tbsp extra virgin olive oil
- salt and pepper

Instructions

2. Place the roast beef, cheese, avocado, scallion, and radishes on a plate.
3. Serve with lettuce, olive oil, mustard, and a hearty dollop of mayonnaise.

Keto tuna plate

Made for: Dinner | **Prep Time:** 10 minutes | **Servings:** 2
Per Serving: Kcal: 930, CARBS 3g, PROTEIN 52g, FAT 76g

Ingredients

- 4 eggs
- 55 g (425 ml) baby spinach
- 280 g tuna in olive oil
- 1 (200 g) avocado
- 120 ml mayonnaise
- ¼ lemon (optional)
- salt and pepper

Instructions

1. Begin by cooking the eggs. Lower them carefully into boiling water and boil for 4-8 minutes, whether you like them soft or hard-boiled.
2. Cool the eggs in ice-cold water for 1-2 minutes when they're done, making it easier to remove the shell.
3. Place eggs, spinach, tuna, and avocado on a plate. Serve with a hearty dollop of mayonnaise and perhaps a wedge of lemon. Season with salt and pepper.

Low-carb pumpkin soup

Made for: Dinner | **Prep Time:** 10 minutes | **Servings:** 1
Per Serving: Kcal: 858, CARBS 14g, PROTEIN 6g, FAT 88g

Ingredients

Pumpkin soup
- ½ (15 g) shallot
- ½ garlic clove
- 70 g pumpkins
- 70 g rutabaga
- ½ tbsp olive oil
- ¼ tsp salt
- 1/8 tsp ground black pepper
- 120 ml vegetable stock
- 55 g butter
- 1/8 lime, the juice

Toppings
- 45 ml mayonnaise or vegan mayonnaise

- 1 tbsp pumpkin seeds, preferably roasted

Instructions

1. Preheat the oven to 400°F (200°C). Peel the pumpkin and cut the flesh into cubes. Do the same with the rutabaga. Peel the shallot and cut it into wedges. Peel the garlic cloves.
2. Put everything in a baking dish. Add olive oil, salt, and pepper.
3. Roast in the oven for 25-30 minutes. Alternatively, you can also fry on medium heat in a large pan until the pumpkin and the turnip is soft.
4. Place the roasted vegetables in a pot. Add vegetable stock or water, and bring to a boil. Let simmer for a couple of minutes. Remove from the stove.
5. Add the butter, divided into cubes. Mix the soup with a hand blender. Add lime juice, herbs, salt, and pepper to taste.
6. Serve the soup with mayonnaise, roasted pumpkin seeds, or our delicious parmesan croutons.

Keto prosciutto-wrapped asparagus with goat cheese

Made for: Dinner | **Prep Time:** 10 minutes | **Servings:** 1
Per Serving: Kcal: 219, CARBS 1g, PROTEIN 11g, FAT 18g

Ingredients

- 3 pieces of green asparagus
- 14 g prosciutto, in thin slices
- 35 g goat cheese
- 1/10 tsp ground black pepper
- ½ tbsp olive oil

Instructions

1. Preheat your oven to 450°F (225°C), preferably with the broiler function.
2. Wash and trim the asparagus.
3. Slice the cheese into as many pieces as asparagus and divide each slice.
4. Cut the slices of prosciutto into two pieces lengthwise and wrap each piece around one asparagus and two pieces of cheese.
5. Place in a baking dish lined with parchment paper. Add pepper and drizzle with olive oil.
6. Broil in the oven for about 15 minutes until golden brown.

Keto lasagna

Lasagna rocks. That enticing flavor mash-up of creamy cheese, hearty tomato sauce, and seasoned ground beef... not to mention garlic and onions. Wait no longer. This keto version is the ultimate comfort food.

Made for: Dinner | **Prep Time:** 15 minutes | **Servings:** 1
Per Serving: Kcal: 752, CARBS 8g, PROTEIN 41g, FAT 60g

Ingredients

Lasagna sheets
- 11/3 eggs, beaten
- 45 g (45 ml) cream cheese
- 1/6 tsp salt
- 13 ml (8 g) ground psyllium husk powder

Meat sauce
- ½ tbsp olive oil
- 1/10 (11 g) yellow onion, finely chopped
- 1/6 garlic clove, finely chopped
- 110 g ground beef or ground turkey
- 1/3 tbsp tomato paste
- 1/10 tbsp dried basil
- 1/6 tsp salt
- 7 ml ground black pepper
- 20 ml water

Cheese topping
- 60 ml sour cream
- 40 ml (19 g) shredded mozzarella cheese
- 20 ml (7 g) shredded Parmesan cheese
- 1/10 tsp salt
- 7 ml ground black pepper
- 20 ml (1.4 g) fresh parsley, finely chopped

Instructions
1. Preheat the oven to 300°F (150°C). Line a baking sheet with parchment paper.
2. In a medium-sized bowl, whisk together the ingredients until a smooth batter. Gradually whisk in the psyllium husk, and then set aside for a few minutes.
3. Add the batter to the center of the parchment paper, and then place another parchment paper on top. Flatten with a rolling pin until the batter is at least 13 x 18" (33 x 45 cm). If you prefer thinner pasta, you can divide the batter into two equal batches, placing it on two baking sheets with parchment paper.
4. Bake each sheet (with parchment paper) for about 10-12 minutes. Set aside to cool. Next, remove the paper and slice pasta into sheets that fit a 9 x 12" (23 x 30 cm) baking dish.

Meat sauce

1. In a large pan, over medium-high heat, warm the olive oil. Add the onion and garlic, stirring until soft. Next, add the beef, tomato paste, and spices, and combine thoroughly until the beef is no longer pink.
2. Add water to the mixture, bring to a boil, lower the heat, and let simmer for at least 15 minutes or until most of the water has evaporated. The sauce should be drier since these lasagna sheets don't soak up as much liquid as traditional ones. Set aside.
3. Preheat the oven to 400°F (200°C). Grease a 9 x 12" (23 x 30 cm) baking dish.

Cheese topping
1. Mix the mozzarella cheese with sour cream and most of the parmesan cheese. Reserve two tablespoons of parmesan cheese for the final topping. Add salt and pepper and stir in the parsley.
2. Alternately layer the pasta sheets and meat sauce in the baking dish, starting with the pasta, followed by the meat sauce.
3. Spread the cheese mixture on the pasta, and finish with the extra parmesan cheese.
4. Bake in the oven for about 30 minutes or until the lasagna has a nicely browned surface. Serve with a green salad and your favorite dressing.

Creamy low-carb broccoli and leek soup

This low-carb soup is the "little black dress" of meals. It can go anywhere and do anything. It can be a lunch or a dinner, an entrée or an appetizer. And it loves, loves, loves extra accouterments, like these cheese chips!

Made for: Dinner | **Prep Time:** 10 minutes | **Servings:** 1
Per Serving: Kcal: 646, CARBS 12g, PROTEIN 21g, FAT 58g

Ingredients

Broccoli soup
- ¼ (22 g) leek
- 70 g (180 ml) head of broccoli
- 180 ml vegetable stock
- 1/10 tsp salt
- 50 g (50 ml) cream cheese
- 60 ml heavy whipping cream
- 1/8 tsp ground black pepper
- 30 ml (5.5 g) fresh basil, chopped
- ¼ garlic clove, pressed

Cheese chips

- 120 ml (55 g) cheddar cheese, or Edam cheese, shredded
- 1/8 tsp paprika powder

Instructions

Broccoli soup

1. Prepare the leek by giving it a quick rinse, patting it dry, and then trimming off the rough, green tips. Slice the remaining leek into thin circles, and discard the root. Next, fill a bowl with cold water and add the sliced leeks. Move them around in the water to remove any remaining dirt or sand, strain, and pat dry.
2. Cut off the core of the broccoli and slice thinly. Divide the rest of the broccoli into smaller florets and reserve.
3. Place the leek and the sliced broccoli core into a medium-size pot. Add the vegetable stock and salt. Cover, and bring to a boil for a few minutes until the broccoli can be easily pierced with a knife.
4. Lower the heat to medium-low, and add the broccoli florets. Simmer for a few minutes until the broccoli is bright green and tender. Add the cream cheese, cream, pepper, basil, and garlic.
5. Blend with an immersion blender until desired consistency. If the soup is too thick, thin it out with water. If you'd like it to have a slightly thicker consistency, add a touch of heavy cream.

Cheese chips

1. Preheat the oven to 400°F (200°C). Line a large, rimmed baking sheet with parchment paper.
2. Place mounds of the shredded cheese by the tablespoon, 1" (2.5 cm) apart, on the parchment paper. Sprinkle each mound with paprika.
3. Bake on the middle rack for about 5-6 minutes or until the cheese has melted. Serve on the side with broccoli and leek soup.

Keto deviled eggs

These amazing keto bites are loaded with flavor and redefine elegance in a small package. They also feature our amazing (if we do say so ourselves) homemade mayonnaise. Serve these for any party or holiday, and be prepared for the rave reviews!

Made for: Dinner | **Prep Time:** 15 minutes | **Servings:** 1
Per Serving: Kcal: 234, CARBS 1g, PROTEIN 14g, FAT 19g

Ingredients

- 2 eggs
- ¼ tsp tabasco
- 15 ml mayonnaise or vegan mayonnaise
- ¼ pinch of herbal salt
- 4 shrimp, cooked and peeled, or strips of smoked salmon
- fresh dill sprigs

Instructions

1. Gently add the eggs to a pot and cover with water, about 2" (5 cm) higher than the eggs. Place the lid on the pot and bring the water to a boil over high heat. Once at a boil, turn off the heat and sit for 8-10 minutes.
2. Remove the eggs from the pot with a slotted spoon, and place them in an ice bath for a few minutes before peeling.
3. Split the eggs in half and scoop out the yolks.
4. Place the egg whites on a plate.
5. In a small bowl, mash the yolks with a fork and add tabasco, herbal salt, and homemade mayonnaise.
6. Add the mixture, using two spoons, to the egg whites and top with a shrimp on each or a piece of smoked salmon.
7. Decorate with dill.

Keto baked salmon with pesto and broccoli

Made for: Dinner | **Prep Time:** 10 minutes | **Servings:** 1
Per Serving: Kcal: 876, CARBS 7g, PROTEIN 54g, FAT 68g

Ingredients

Green pesto sauce

- 1 tbsp green pesto
- 30 ml mayonnaise or vegan mayonnaise
- 40 ml (30 g) full-fat Greek yogurt (4% fat)
- salt and pepper, to taste

Salmon and broccoli

- 220 g salmon, boneless fillets
- 1 tbsp green pesto
- salt and pepper, to taste
- 110 g (290 ml) broccoli

Instructions

1. Place the salmon skin-side down in a greased baking dish. Spread pesto on top, and salt and pepper to taste. Spread out the broccoli around it.
2. Bake in the oven at 350°F (175°C) for about 20 minutes, or until the salmon flakes easily with a fork.

3. Meanwhile, stir the pesto sauce ingredients together and refrigerate.
4. To serve, plate the salmon with the pesto sauce and enjoy!

Smoked ham stuffed zucchini boats

Ham, herbs, and cheese anchor a low-carb filling that carries zucchini from yum to YOWSA. Familiar, satisfying, and oh-so-delicious. If you like zucchini, we promise this dish will float your boat.

Made for: Dinner | **Prep Time:** 10 minutes | **Servings:** 1
Per Serving: Kcal: 537, CARBS 8g, PROTEIN 33g, FAT 41g

Ingredients
- 190 g zucchini
- ¼ tsp salt
- ¼ tbsp olive oil
- 100 g smoked deli ham
- 28 g (32 ml) cottage cheese
- ½ tbsp mayonnaise
- ½ tbsp red onions, finely chopped
- 1/8 tbsp dried rosemary
- 90 ml (45 g) cheddar cheese, shredded
- salt and pepper

For serving
- 50 g (325 ml) lettuce
- 1 tbsp olive oil
- 1/8 tbsp white wine vinegar
- salt and pepper

Instructions
1. Preheat the oven to 400°F (200°C).
2. Split each zucchini in half, lengthwise, and remove the seeds. Sprinkle with salt and let sit for 10 minutes.
3. Blot off the drops of liquid with paper towels. Place the halves in a greased baking dish.
4. Chop the ham coarsely and mix with cottage cheese, mayonnaise, red onion, and spices. Add a third of the grated cheese. Salt and pepper to taste.
5. Distribute the mixture into the zucchini halves and sprinkle the remaining cheese on top. Bake for approximately 20–30 minutes or until the zucchini boats have turned a nice golden color.
6. Mix oil, vinegar, salt, and pepper into a simple vinaigrette. Serve the zucchini boats beside a simple salad made with lettuce and vinaigrette.

Cod loin with horseradish and browned butter

Cod loin with horseradish and browned butter is a truly classic Swedish combo. Scandinavian elegance and simplicity come together in this authentic keto dish that you can prepare in no time and hopefully will love as much as we do.

Made for: Dinner | **Prep Time:** 10 minutes | **Servings:** 1
Per Serving: Kcal: 435, CARBS 7g, PROTEIN 33g, FAT 30g

Ingredients
- 170 g cod, boneless fillets
- ¼ tsp salt
- 21 g fresh horseradish, grated
- 35 g butter
- 110 g fresh green beans
- salt and pepper
- 7 g celery root, finely sliced (optional)

Instructions
1. Salt fish pieces and keep them in the refrigerator for an hour. If you don't have enough time, you can salt and fry the fish straight away, but first, start with peeling and grating the horseradish.
2. Wipe the fish completely dry with paper towels. Heat one-third of the butter and fry fish on medium heat for 3-4 minutes on each side. Baste the fish with the butter in the pan now and then to prevent drying out.
3. Reduce the heat towards the end. Season with freshly ground pepper. Remove from the pan when just cooked through to ensure a nice, flaky result.
4. Melt the rest of the butter in a saucepan on medium heat and keep heating until it gets a nutty fragrance and lights brown color.
5. Boil beans in salted water for a few minutes.
6. Place the fish on a bed of freshly cooked beans. Drizzle browned butter on the fish and top with freshly grated horseradish.

Grilled white fish with zucchini and kale pesto

Made for: Dinner | **Prep Time:** 10 minutes | **Servings:** 1
Per Serving: Kcal: 648, CARBS 5g, PROTEIN 37g, FAT5 3g

Ingredients

Kale pesto
- 21 g kale

- ¾ tbsp lemon juice or lime juice
- 14 g (33 ml) walnuts
- ¼ garlic clove
- 1/8 tsp salt
- 1/10 tsp ground black pepper
- 30 ml olive oil

Fish and zucchini
- 140 g zucchini
- ¼ tbsp lemon juice
- 1/8 tsp salt
- ½ tbsp olive oil
- 170 g white fish fillets (for example, cod, halibut, flounder, or Alaskan whitefish)
- 1/10 tsp ground black pepper

Instructions

1. Start preparing the pesto by chopping the kale roughly. Place the kale, walnuts, lime, and garlic in a blender or food processor, and purée until smooth. Season with salt and pepper. Add the oil towards the end and process a bit more. Set aside.
2. Rinse the zucchini and cut thinly with a sharp knife, slicer, or mandolin. Put the slices in a bowl. Season with salt and pepper to taste, and dress with lemon juice and olive oil. Set aside.
3. Salt both sides of the fish and let sit for a few minutes. Wipe off excess liquid and brush with oil.
4. Grill or fry the fish for a few minutes on each side in a frying pan with oil. Season with pepper and serve together with the zucchini and pesto.

Spicy shrimp salad

Turn up the heat with this keto shrimp salad. Hot cooked shrimp served over a bed of spinach with smooth avocado and crunchy cucumber. It's the perfect salad combined with a delicious ginger and garlic dressing.

Made for: Dinner | **Prep Time:** 10 minutes | **Servings:** 1
Per Serving: Kcal: 592, CARBS 8g, PROTEIN 24g, FAT 50g

Ingredients

Ginger dressing
- 30 ml light olive oil or avocado oil
- ½ tbsp minced, fresh ginger
- ¼ lime, juice
- ¼ tbsp tamari soy sauce
- ¼ garlic clove, pressed
- salt and pepper, to taste

Salad
- ½ (100 g) avocado

- ¼ lime, juice
- 70 g cucumber, peeled, cut in half lengthwise, seeded, and sliced
- 28 g (220 ml) baby spinach
- sea salt, for seasoning

Shrimp
- ½ tbsp olive oil for frying
- ½ garlic clove, pressed
- 1 tsp chilli powder
- 140 g fresh shrimp, peeled, deveined
- salt and pepper

For Serving
- 1 tsp chopped fresh cilantro
- 1 tbsp chopped hazelnuts or salted peanuts (optional)

Instructions

Ginger dressing
1. Add the Ginger dressing ingredients to a small bowl. Using an immersion blender, mix over low speed until combined. Set aside.

Salad
2. Slice the avocado in half, and remove the pit. Using a spoon, scoop out the avocado flesh, and cut it into slices. Place in a small bowl, and stir together with the lime juice.
3. Arrange the spinach, avocado, and cucumber slices on a serving platter or large plate. Season with the sea salt, and set aside.

Shrimp
1. Heat the olive oil in a medium-sized pan over medium heat. Stir in the garlic and chilli powder. Add the shrimp, stir to combine, and fry for a couple of minutes per side until the shrimp are pink and cooked through, be careful not to overcook, or the shrimp may be rubbery. Pre-cooked shrimp should only be heated for 1 - 2 minutes. Season with salt and pepper to taste.
2. Use a slotted spoon to place the shrimp, with some of the spicy sauce, on top of the vegetables. For serving, sprinkle the nuts and cilantro on top, drizzled with the ginger dressing.

Broccoli cheddar soup

Creamy, cheesy comfort in a bowl, cheddar soup is your name! It's not only low carb but quick and super easy to whip up from scratch. This velvety smooth soup will warm you up from top to toe, satisfaction guaranteed.

Made for: Dinner | **Prep Time:** 10 minutes | **Servings:** 1
Per Serving: Kcal: 333, CARBS7g, PROTEIN8g, FAT30g

Ingredients

- 75 g (200 ml) broccoli
- 1/6 tbsp olive oil
- 9 g butter
- 1/6 (18 g) red onion, roughly chopped
- ½ garlic clove, chopped
- 1/10 tsp salt
- 7 ml ground black pepper
- 1/10 tsp paprika powder
- 1/6 pinch cayenne pepper
- 80 ml chicken broth or water
- 40 ml heavy whipping cream
- 40 ml (19 g) cheddar cheese, shredded

Instructions

1. Clean and cut the broccoli and separate the florets from the stalk. Roughly chop the stalks and cut the florets into small pieces.
2. Heat the olive oil with one-third of the butter in a pot or a saucepan. When melted, add the roughly chopped onion and the broccoli stalks. Fry on medium heat until they start to brown. Add garlic cloves and keep frying until lightly browned.
3. Season with salt, pepper, paprika, and cayenne pepper. Combine well and cook for another minute.
4. Add broth and stir well. Cover and let simmer for 5 minutes.
5. Transfer the cooked vegetables and broth into a food processor and pulse until the ingredients are smooth and creamy soup.
6. Heat the rest of the butter in the same pot and fry the broccoli florets. Stir the broccoli only occasionally to get a lovely roasted flavor.
7. Pour the blended soup mixture through a sieve into the pot. For a chunkier soup, you can skip the sieve. Combine well and add more salt and pepper if needed. If the soup seems too thick, add some water or broth.
8. Allow the mixture to simmer for a few minutes.
9. Add cream and cheese and mix well. Cook until the cheese has melted.
10. Serve hot and garnish with some shredded cheddar cheese.

South Indian Egg Curry

Made for: Lunch | **Prep Time:** 10 minutes | **Servings:** 4
Per Serving: Kcal: 245, Carbs (net) 7.1 grams, Protein 13.8 grams, Fat 17.4 grams

Ingredients

- 8 Hardboiled Large Eggs
- 30ml/g Coconut Oil (we use cooking coconut oil, which has no taste or smell - we use this one)
- 1.5 tsp Mustard Seeds
- 1.5 tbsp Kaffir Lime Leaves (fresh or dried - we used 4 dried leaves)
- 100g Shallots, finely chopped
- 50g ginger, peeled and finely chopped
- 1/2 tsp Ground Turmeric
- 1/2 tsp Kashmiri Chilli Powder
- 400g Tinned Chopped Tomatoes
- 250ml Vegetable Stock (we use Bouillon)
- 1/2 tsp Salt
- 1/2 tsp Truvia / Natvia / Pure Via Sweetener
- Small bunch of coriander, chopped

Directions

1. Heat the oil in a large saucepan over medium/high heat.
2. Add the mustard seeds to the oil. Allow them to pop - you may find a splatter guard useful here!
3. After a few minutes, add the chopped shallots, ginger, and kaffir lime leaves (tear/crush these). Combine over medium heat.
4. Allow cooking for 5-10 minutes until golden.
5. Add the turmeric and chilli, followed by the tin of chopped tomatoes. Combine and allow to simmer for 10 minutes on low heat.
6. Add the stock, salt, and sweetener. Stir, rest the hardboiled eggs in the curry and simmer for 10-15 minutes.
7. Season with salt & pepper and top with chopped coriander to finish.

Pork Recipes

BBQ Pulled Pork

Pork Recipes | **Prep Time:** 10 minutes | **Servings:** 4
Per Serving: Kcal: 329, Carbs (net) 5 grams, Protein 43 grams,
Fat 15 grams

Ingredients
- 1 small (around 750g) Boneless Pork Joint (or 500g Skinless Pork Loin)
- 15ml Olive Oil

BBQ Sauce
- 20g Butter / Olive Oil
- 100g Shallots, finely diced
- 400g Tinned Chopped Tomatoes / Passata
- 2 Garlic Cloves, finely chopped (or 5g Garlic Puree)
- 2 tsp Smoked Paprika or 2 tsp Ketoroma BBQ Blend
- 1/4 tsp Hot Chilli Powder
- 30ml Apple Cider Vinegar
- 10g Truvia / Natvia / Pure Via Sweetener or 1-2 Monkfruit Sweetener Drops

Directions
1. Preheat the oven to 170°C.
2. Heat the 15ml olive oil in a large pan and sear the pork on all sides. Transfer this to an ovenproof dish while you make the sauce.
3. Heat the 20g butter/olive oil in a saucepan and fry the onions & garlic for 2-3 minutes to soften but not brown. Add the tomatoes/passata, spices, vinegar, and sweetener, and bring to a boil.
4. Reduce the heat, cover with a lid and allow to cook for 8-10 minutes. If you want to make a smooth sauce, allow this to cool before either blending in a jug blender or using a stick blender.
5. Pour the sauce around the pork, cover tightly with foil, and bake for 90-120 minutes. If using the pork loin, you may need to add a little extra liquid to prevent the sauce from drying out.
6. Remove the foil. If you've used a joint with skin, remove this by running a knife between skin & meat and place it on another baking tray to a crisp in the oven.
7. Using a couple of forks, break the meat apart and spoon the sauce over the meat. You can return the dish to the oven to reduce the sauce slightly.

BBQ Sauce & Marinade

Pork Recipes | **Prep Time:** 10 minutes | **Servings:** 2
Per Serving: Kcal: 59, Carbs (net) 4.2 grams, Protein 1.5 grams, Fat 4 grams

Ingredients
- 20g Butter / 20ml Olive Oil
- 100g Shallots, finely diced
- 2 Garlic Cloves, finely chopped, or 5g Garlic Puree
- 400g Tin Chopped Tomatoes / Passata (no added sugars)
- 2 tsp Smoked Paprika
- 1/4 tsp Cayenne Pepper
- 30ml Apple Cider Vinegar
- 10g Truvia / Natvia / Pure Via Sweetener

Directions
1. Heat the oil/butter in a saucepan and fry the onions & garlic for 2-3 minutes to soften but not brown.
2. Add the tomatoes/passata, spices, vinegar, and sweetener. Bring to the boil.
3. Reduce the heat, cover with a lid, and allow to cook for 8-10 minutes.
4. If you want to make a smooth sauce, allow this to cool before either blending in a jug blender or using a stick blender.

Marinade: Ribs
1. Place the ribs into a large food bag and spoon the mix over the meat - per 500g of meat, you will need around 100g of sauce. Squeeze the air out of the bag, seal the top and then massage the sauce into the meat carefully, so you don't puncture the bag.
2. Allow the meat to marinate overnight and roast the rack in the oven at 160°C for around 45-50 minutes.

Bolognese Base recipe

Pork Recipes | **Prep Time:** 15 minutes | **Servings:** 4
Per Serving: Kcal: 364, 5.4 g Carbs, 24.4g Protein, 24.4g Fat

Ingredients
- 30g Olive Oil
- 75g Bacon, chopped small
- 100g Leeks, chopped small
- 50g Carrots, chopped small
- 100g Celery, chopped small
- 1tsp Oregano or Mixed Herbs
- 3 Garlic cloves or 1 1/2 tsp garlic powder
- 1 tsp Ketoroma Curry Blend - not enough to taste it, but enough to give an edge :-)
- 500g Beef mince (I like 250g pork & 250g Beef)

- 400g Tinned tomatoes
- 200g Coldwater, to rinse out the tinned tomatoes and add to the pan
- 1tsp Salt
- Freshly ground pepper
- 15g 85% Dark Chocolate (this is included in the macros, but it is optional - it makes the meat sauce a lot richer)
- 15g Basil, to decorate

Directions

1. Add the olive oil to a large non-stick saucepan and gently heat.
2. Add the chopped bacon, leeks, carrots & celery and cook for about 5 minutes until softened.
3. Add the garlic, herbs, curry blend, and meat to the saucepan. Carry on frying until the meat has browned, for around 5 - 10 minutes.
4. Add the tinned tomatoes, water (I use the water to clean out the tomato tins), salt & pepper.
5. Now simmer for about 30 - 45 minutes, or until you're happy that the sauce has reduced to a beautiful, silky sauce
6. Stir in the dark chocolate chunks until melted.
7. And finally, top with basil leaves, or sprinkle on when serving.

Bubble & Squeak

Pork Recipes | **Prep Time:** 15 minutes | **Servings:** 4
Per Serving: Kcal: 184, 8.1g Carbs, 12.4g Fat, 9.6g Protein

Ingredients

- 300g Diced Swede - Par Boiled for around 10 minutes or until soft.
- 200g Leftover Veggies, e.g., a combination of cabbage, sprouts, broccoli
- 100g Shallots - chopped
- 150g Bacon, cut into thin strips
- 20g Butter / 20ml Olive Oil
- Seasoning - Salt & Pepper
- Optional - Handful of Fresh Sage Leaves, roughly chopped

Directions

1. Heat the butter/oil in a large frying pan over medium heat.
2. Add the shallots and chopped bacon and fry for 3 - 5 minutes to soften.
3. Add the leftover veggies and the sage, combine with the shallots and allow to cook through for 2 - 3 minutes.

4. Add the diced swede, combine it with the rest of the pan, and use a masher to work around the pan to push the mix together.
5. Keep the heat low/medium to prevent the dish from burning, but you aim to create a nice golden color.
6. You can transfer the mix into an ovenproof dish and bake for 10-15 minutes or serve from the pan.

Bulgarian Sarmi

Pork Recipes | **Prep Time:** 20 minutes | **Servings:** 4
Per Serving: Kcal: 312, Carbs (net) 8.5 grams, Protein 28 grams, Fat 17 grams

Ingredients

- 1 medium Whole White Cabbage
- 20ml Olive Oil (or 20g Butter)
- 100g Leeks, finely chopped
- 100g Shallots, finely chopped
- 500g Pork Mince (10-12% Fat)
- 100g Carrots, grated
- 2 tsp Smoked Paprika
- 10g Fresh Parsley
- 200ml Vegetable Stock

Directions

1. Add 200-300ml water to a saucepan and bring to a boil.
2. Remove any limp outer leaves and the core from the cabbage. Place the whole cabbage in the saucepan.
3. Cover and reduce the heat to gently simmer for 5 minutes. Lift the whole cabbage out and allow it to cool.
4. Heat the oil/butter in a frying pan and gently fry the leeks & shallots for 3-5 minutes. Either remove them from the pan or push them to the side and add the pork.
5. Fry the pork over medium /high heat for 3-5 minutes using a spatula to break up the mince to ensure it cooks evenly.
6. Re-add the leeks/shallots, and then add the carrots & paprika. Fry over medium heat, add half the parsley, and season with salt & pepper - fry for a couple more minutes. Allow cooling.
7. While the meat is cooling, start to remove around 12 leaves from the cabbage.
8. Spoon some mix into each leaf and roll into a little parcel. You'll be surprised how flexible and robust the leaves will be!
9. Lay the parcels in a large pan and add the stock. Put the pan over high heat to boil, then reduce the heat to low and cover with a lid. Simmer for 15-20 minutes.

10. Sprinkle the remaining parsley on top and serve with a rich tomato sauce!

Chicken, Bacon & Asparagus Salad

Pork Recipes | **Prep Time:** 5 minutes | **Servings:** 1
Per Serving: Kcal: 341, Carbs (net) 1.8 grams, Protein 31.8 grams, Fat 23.6 grams

Ingredients
- 100g Chicken Breast
- 2 Rashers of Bacon
- 80g Asparagus
- Optional: 10g Parmesan Cheese, grated
- 15ml Olive Oil
- Handful of spinach

Directions
1. Heat the oil in a frying pan/wok over gentle heat.
2. Add the chicken and brown it on all sides. Allow cooking over medium heat for 5 minutes.
3. Move the chicken to the side of the pan and add the bacon. Fry for 1-2 minutes.
4. Add the asparagus.
5. Allow to cook for 2-3 minutes or until the asparagus is cooked to your taste.
6. Serve on a bed of spinach and serve with the parmesan cheese (optional).

Chicken & Chorizo

Pork Recipes | **Prep Time:** 25 minutes | **Servings:** 4
Per Serving: Kcal: 563, 13g Carbs, 50.8g Protein, 33.6g Fat

Ingredients
- Follow the recipe for Rice Base Dish
- 20g Olive oil
- 400g Chicken breast - chunky chopped
- 250g Chorizo - chunky chopped
- 120g Red Pepper - chunky chopped
- 2 tsp Paprika
- 25g Fresh, flat-leaf parsley, roughly chopped
- Salt & pepper

Directions
1. Follow the instructions for the Rice Base Dish
2. Oven 180C, Ninja 170C, or this can be fried in a non-stick frying pan
3. Add chicken, chorizo, peppers, olive oil, paprika, and seasoning to a bowl. Give it a good mix
4. Pop on the oven for about 25 - 30 minutes or until the chicken is cooked

5. Once cooked, add all the ingredients, including the fresh parsley, to the Rice Base recipe and stir through
6. This can be quickly stir-fried to reheat the rice dish or popped into the fridge
7. To reheat, either stir fry or microwave. If reheating in the oven, make sure you cover the dish with foil so it doesn't dry out
8. Enjoy:

Creamy Chicken & Ham Pie

Pork Recipes | **Prep Time:** 15 minutes | **Servings:** 4
Per Serving: Kcal: 1346, 14g Carbs, 77g Protein, 108g Fat

Ingredients
Pie Crust
- 1 batch Pie Crust (follow this link to take you to the recipe)

The Filling
- 400g Chicken - Small, roughly chopped
- 200g Cooked Ham or Gammon - Small, roughly chopped
- 300g Leeks - Small, roughly chopped
- 20g Butter
- 20g Olive oil
- 1/2 tsp garlic
- 250ml Milk
- 150ml Double Cream
- 1 Chicken stock cube
- 20g Parmesan
- 20g Arrowroot (mixed with about 30ml water to create a thickening agent)
- Salt & Pepper (I added 1/2 tsp salt & 1/4 tsp pepper)

Directions

Pie Crust
1. 1 batch Pie Crust (follow this link to take you to the recipe)

The Filling
1. Add the butter & Olive oil to a large pan and fry the leeks for about 5 - 10 minutes, until it's softened but not browned (almost translucent)
2. Now add the chicken & fry until cooked (about 5 - 10 minutes)
3. Add all the remaining ingredients APART from the arrowroot mixed with water, stir well and bring up to almost bubbling and turn down to a gentle simmer

4. Now add the arrowroot and stir through the sauce in the pan. Allow thickening. If you'd like it a little thicker, add more arrowroot, mixed with a little water in the same way. Or, if you'd like to keep the carbs lower, add a sprinkling of ready grated mozzarella & stir through until it thickens
5. Now pour into your prepared Pie Crust base and go back to the Pie Crust recipe and instruction no.8 onwards

Chinese - Style Belly Pork & Dip

Pork Recipes | **Prep Time:** 10 minutes | **Servings:** 4
Per Serving: Kcal: 758, 5.8g Carbs, 63.4g Protein, 52.4g Fat

Ingredients
- 750g - 1kg Belly Pork
- 2-3 tsp Ketoroma Chinese Blend (link here)
- 60ml Water
- 200ml Stock - preferably homemade chicken or pork stock. A stock cube will add around 2g carbs to the dish
- 30ml Liquid Aminos
- 15g Tomato Puree or 30g Passata
- 1/2 tsp Truvia / Natvia / Pure Via Sweetener

Directions
PREP

1. Cut the belly pork into bite-sized chunks and place them in a food bag.
2. Mix the Chinese Blend with the water and add to the belly pork.
3. Allow to marinate for several hours or preferably overnight.

COOKING

1. Add the stock to a large pan, bring to a boil and add the belly pork.
2. Bring back to the boil, reduce heat and cover with a well-fitting lid.
3. Allow cooking for 45-60 mins gently. Ensure the pan does not dry out.
4. Transfer the belly pork to a roasting tray (or air crisping basket using a Ninja Foodi / Grill), leaving the sauce in the pan.
5. Roast at 220°C (Air Crisp at 200°C in the Ninja) for 15-25 minutes, depending on how crunchy you want the meat/crackling.
6. While the belly pork is cooking, bring the sauce to a boil and add the liquid aminos and sweetener.
7. Mix well and reduce to your preferred texture. The sauce will naturally thicken from cooking the belly pork in it.

Cooked Breakfast

Pork Recipes | **Prep Time:** 10 minutes | **Servings:** 4
Per Serving: Kcal: 394, Carbs (net) 3 grams, Protein 21.2 grams, Fat 32.1 grams

Ingredients
- 2 Rashers of Bacon
- 60g (1/2 medium) Avocado
- 1 Large Egg
- 70g Closed Cup Mushrooms
- 30g Spinach
- 10g Butter or Cooking Coconut Oil

Directions
1. Melt the butter/oil on medium heat and fry the bacon in a large pan.
2. Add the mushrooms.
3. Add the egg and sliced avocado if the pan is big enough once the bacon is almost cooked. If not, wait until it is fully cooked, remove the bacon & mushrooms from the pan, and keep them warm while cooking your egg and avocado.
4. Cook the egg to your preference and lightly brown the avocado.
5. Serve on a bed of spinach.

Keto Crackslaw

Pork Recipes | **Prep Time:** 5 minutes | **Servings:** 2
Per Serving: Kcal: 377, Carbs (net) 8 grams, Protein 30.8 grams, Fat 22 grams

Ingredients
- 30g Unsalted Butter or 30ml Olive Oil
- 400g Hard Cabbage (white or red), sliced
- 80g Shallots, chopped
- 10ml White Wine Vinegar
- 1/2 tsp Garlic Puree
- 1/4 tsp Chilli Flakes
- 250g Lean Pork Mince (5% fat)
- 2 tsp Sesame Seeds
- Salt & Pepper

Directions
1. Heat the butter/oil in a large pan/wok and add the cabbage & onion. Fry for around 5 minutes over medium heat. Don't let the cabbage brown.
2. Add all spices and vinegar and cook for 1-2 minutes, still on medium heat.
3. Put the cabbage in a bowl, return the pan to heat, and add the pork. Turn the heat up high.
4. Fry the pork until brown throughout, and then add the cabbage mix to the meat. Bring back to full heat.

5. Add salt, pepper, and sesame seeds, and serve.

Fried Sprouts & Bacon

Pork Recipes | **Prep Time:** 10 minutes | **Servings:** 4
Per Serving: Kcal: 128, Carbs (net) 4.2 grams, Protein 6.8 grams, Fat 9.6 grams

Ingredients

- 20g Butter
- 200g Brussel Sprouts
- 4 Rashers of Bacon, cut into strips
- 2 Garlic Cloves, finely chopped
- Optional: 1/4 tsp Kashmiri Chilli
- Optional: 20g Flaked Almonds

Directions

1. Trim any outer leaves that are needed to be removed and place in a large pan of boiling, salted water. Bring the pan back to a boil, reduce the heat and allow to cook over a gentle heat for 5 minutes. Drain the water.
2. If you are using the sprouts straight away, leave them in a colander. If you finish the dish off at a later point, plunge the sprouts into a pan of cold water to prevent them from over-cooking.
3. In a large frying pan, melt the butter over medium heat. Add the garlic and bacon and fry for 8-10 minutes.
4. Add the sprouts to the pan and combine with the bacon & garlic. If you're adding the chilli & almonds, add these in now.
5. If you are heating the sprouts from cold, cover the pan with a lid, reduce the heat and allow it to heat fully - this takes around 5 minutes.

Paella (Haddock & Chorizo)

Pork Recipes | **Prep Time:** 10 minutes | **Servings:** 4
Per Serving: Kcal: 367, 11.4g Carbs, 37.4g Protein, 16.4g Fat

Ingredients
- 30ml Olive Oil
- 100g Shallots, finely sliced
- 3 Garlic Cloves, finely sliced
- 100g Red Bell Pepper, finely sliced
- 60g Chorizo, diced
- 800g Cauliflower
- 200ml Stock (chicken / fish) or water
- 2 tsp Smoked Paprika
- 1 tsp Pink Himalayan / Rock Salt
- 1/2 - 1 tsp Chilli Flakes
- A handful of Fresh Flat Leaf Parsley, finely chopped (save some for topping)
- 200g Passata

- 600g Haddock Fillets (skinless)
- Salt & Pepper

Directions
1. Heat the olive oil in a large pan over low heat.
2. Add the shallots, garlic, pepper, and chorizo. Allow the veg to soften and the oil from the chorizo to seep out.
3. Meanwhile, break the cauliflower into florets and blitz in a food processor until it resembles rice.
4. By this point, the oil in the bottom of the pan should be orange. Add the cauliflower rice and combine with the veg & chorizo.
5. Add the stock/water to the pan, the passata, smoked paprika, salt, chilli flakes, and parsley. Cover the pan with a lid for a few minutes.
6. Remove the lid, give the rice a quick mix, and lay the fish on top (break this into large chunks - some will flake as the dish cooks). Cover the pan with a lid again.
7. After 6 - 8 minutes, remove the lid and carefully combine the fish with the rice. Season to taste and serve.

Keto Jerk Ribs

Pork Recipes | **Prep Time:** 30 minutes | **Servings:** 4
Per Serving: Kcal: 411, Carbs (net) 1.7 grams, Protein 35.1 grams, Fat 28.6 grams

Ingredients
Ribs

- 4 x 500g Racks of Pork Ribs
- 2 tsp Pink Himalayan / Rock / Sea Salt

Marinade
- 30g Coconut Oil, melted, or 30ml Olive Oil
- 100g Shallots, grated or finely diced
- 2-3 Garlic Cloves, grated or finely diced (or 1 tsp Garlic Puree)
- 2 tbsp Allspice Berries
- 2 tsp Dried Thyme
- 1 tsp Ground Nutmeg
- 1 tsp Ground Cinnamon
- 1 tsp Chilli Flakes
- 1 tsp Pink Himalayan / Rock / Sea Salt
- 1 tsp Black Peppercorns / Ground Pepper
- Optional: 1 Scotch Bonnet Pepper - this is one of the hottest chilies in the world, so use a little or half to start with, and discard the seeds to reduce the heat if required.

Directions

1. Put the pork ribs in a large pan, cover with cold water, and add salt.
2. Bring to the boil, reduce the heat and simmer for 45 minutes.
3. Remove the ribs from the water and allow them to cool.
4. While the ribs are cooling, prepare the marinade.
5. In a bowl, mix all of the marinade ingredients into a paste. You could use a small food processor to create a smoother paste.
6. Once the ribs are cool, choose to cut them into individual ribs or leave them on a rack.
7. Cover the ribs in the paste but keep a little back to add partway through cooking.
8. Place the ribs on a baking tray (or BBQ) and cook for 30 minutes at 190-200°C.
9. During the cooking process, apply the remaining marinade.

Keto Pierogi with Bacon & Cheddar

Pork Recipes | **Prep Time:** 10 minutes | **Servings:** 4
Per Serving: Kcal: 813, 13g Carbs, 39g Protein, 67g Fat

Ingredients
- 400g Cauliflower
- 240g Ground Almonds
- 170g Grated Mozzarella
- 120g Cheddar
- 100g Bacon
- 60g Soured Cream
- 1 Egg Yolk
- 30g Butter (15g for the cauliflower and 15g for the pastry)
- 30g Fresh Parsley
- 0.5 tsp Salt
- 1 tsp Onion Powder
- 0.5 tsp Xanthan Gum
- 0.5 tsp Garlic Powder
- 0.5 tsp Black Pepper

Directions

The Filling

1. Take a double boiler and fill the bottom pot with an inch of water. Bring it to a boil with a tight-fitting lid. Heat a skillet on medium heat, fry the bacon until crisp, and then set aside on a paper towel to drain. Keep the bacon grease in the skillet.

2. Wash and trim the cauliflower, chop it into small florets and then add it to the steamer section of the double boiler. Steam for 10 minutes until just fork tender.

3. Empty the water from the bottom pot, dump the cauliflower into the bottom pot, top it with the butter, and then the lid so that the butter can melt. Mince the parsley and crisp bacon, then grate the cheddar cheese with the small side of a cheese grater. Once the butter has melted, use a blender to puree the cauliflower until smooth. Stir in the sour cream and half the onion powder, garlic powder, salt, and pepper. Add the parsley, bacon, and cheddar until fully combined, then set aside.

The Dough

1. Add the almond flour, onion powder, garlic powder, sea salt, and xanthan gum to the safe microwave bowl, then whisk until fully combined. Grate the mozzarella, toss almond flour, and plop the butter right on top.

2. Microwave for 60 seconds, stir, and then microwave for an additional 30 seconds. Stir well, being sure the cheese has fully melted, then knead in the egg yolk. Divide the dough into 12 equal portions.

3. Set a large piece of wax paper aside for the finished pierogies.

4. Roll a portion of dough into a ball and then place it between two pieces of wax paper. Roll it out into a circle, nice and thin, about 3.5 " wide, then remove the top piece of wax paper. Place 1 – 1 ½ TBSP of the filling into the circle's center. Use the wax paper to fold the circle in half to create a pierogi. Push the edges together to seal and then remove from the wax paper and set aside. Repeat for each ball of dough.

To Finish

1. Heat a skillet on medium heat with extra butter or the bacon grease. Fry sliced onion, if desired, and then add the Keto Pierogies to the hot skillet. Fry until the bottom is golden, about 3-5 minutes, and then flip them over and do the same with the other side. Serve hot with sour cream and fried onions if desired.

Leek & Ham Cheesy Bake

Pork Recipes | **Prep Time:** 10 minutes | **Servings:** 4
Per Serving: Kcal: 242, 2.5g Carbs, 12.1g Protein, 19.6g Fat

Ingredients
- 170g Leeks - chunky chopped
- 125g Ready cooked and sliced ham - I like diced up gammon in this dish

The Sauce
- 100ml Milk
- 50g Double cream
- 30g Cream Cheese
- 30g Ready grated Mozerella
- 1/2 tsp Mustard Powder
- S & P

Topping
- 1/2 90 sec bread
- Seasoning
- 50g Grated cheddar

Directions
2. Oven 180C
3. Ovenproof dish, lightly grease
4. Cut your leeks into strips that will fit the base of your ovenproof dish (lol, or slice anyway that you like :-))
5. Steam or boil the leeks until cooked and fill the base of your ovenproof dish
6. Break the cooked ham into pieces and scatter over the leeks

The Sauce
1. Meanwhile, add all the sauce ingredients to a non-stick saucepan
2. Bring the sauce to almost boiling, and then turn it down to a gentle simmer. Keep stirring until the sauce thickens
3. Pour over the ham and leeks

Final toppings
1. Whiz up your bread to crumbs and season
2. Sprinkle all over the sauce
3. Now sprinkle over the grated cheddar
4. Bake for about 15 - 20 minutes

Lorne Sausage

Pork Recipes | **Prep Time:** 10 minutes | **Servings:** 4
Per Serving: Kcal: 278, 0.4g Carbs, 31.5g Protein, 17.8g Fat

Ingredients

90 Second Bread / Breadcrumbs
- 35g Milled Linseed or Ground Almonds
- 1 Egg
- 1/2 tsp Baking Powder
- Seasoning

The Sausage
- Breadcrumbs - See the above ingredients
- 250g Beef Mince
- 250g Pork Mince
- 75g Water
- 1/2 tsp Nutmeg
- 1/2 tsp Coriander (dried or fresh)
- 1 tsp salt
- Pepper
- A sprinkling of Kashmiri chilli - Optional extra (requested by my husband!)

Directions

Breadcrumbs
1. Add all the bread ingredients to a small bowl and mix well
2. Pop in the microwave for 1 minute, or until completely cooked
3. Slice so you can toast it, then toast till lightly browned
4. Allow to cool slightly, then whiz up in a Bullet, hand blender, or food processor

The Sausage
1. Line a large baking tray with greaseproof paper - you are not going to cook in this tray, but it will need to go in the freezer
2. In a large bowl, mix both of your meats till they are well combined
3. A tip from The Spice Guy, push all the meat up around the side of the bowl; please refer to the picture
4. Now add all the ingredients to the well in the meat (including the breadcrumbs)
5. If you can, get your hands in and mix everything until all the water and seasonings are mixed evenly throughout the mix
6. Press the mixture into the lined baking tray. Push it in as tightly as possible to ensure there are no gaps in the mix
7. Once all packed down in the tin, score 12 sausages, please refer to the picture, cover with cling film, and pop in the freezer for an hour *
8. Once frozen, break up into 12 slices
9. You can either pop these into a container and put them back into the freezer (pop a little greaseproof paper between each slice to stop them sticking) and cook from frozen, or defrost the night before for a quicker cook

Cooking instructions
1. If the sausages are already defrosted, shallow fry. Only a tiny bit of oil is needed
2. Cook on medium heat for about 4 minutes on each side, until well browned on both sides and cooked through

Pancetta & Chilli Courgetti

Pork Recipes | **Prep Time:** 10 minutes | **Servings:** 2
Per Serving: Kcal: 479, Carbs (net) 10 grams, Protein 23 grams, Fat 34 grams

Ingredients
- 20g Butter
- 2-3 Garlic Cloves, finely chopped
- 20g Fresh Red Chilli, finely chopped
- 80g Baby Plum / Cherry Tomatoes
- 170g Smoked Pancetta
- 200g Leeks, sliced into thin strips
- 400g Courgetti (not whole courgettes) - see description above for details.
- 20g Parmesan Cheese

Directions
1. See the description above for details on how we make the courgette.
2. Add the butter to a large frying pan and melt over medium heat. Add the garlic, chilli, tomatoes, and pancetta.
3. Cook for 5-6 minutes over medium heat to soften and let the flavors combine.
4. Once the tomatoes have softened, layer the leeks and courgette on top and turn the heat up to full.
5. Cook over high heat for 2-3 minutes. Don't over-cook this!
6. Sprinkle with parmesan and serve :)

Pancetta and Leek Stuffing

Pork Recipes | **Prep Time:** 10 minutes | **Servings:** 10
Per Serving: Kcal: 132, Carbs (net) 1.2 grams, Fat 11 grams, Protein 6.4 grams

Ingredients
- 90 Second Bread
- 1 Large Egg
- 1/2 tsp Baking Powder
- 40g Pine Nuts
- 200g Celery
- 200g Leeks
- 200g Pancetta (smoked or unsmoked)
- 1 tsp Dried Thyme

Directions
1. First, make a 90-second bread by following the recipe (click here). This can also be replaced with 100g of Megga bread.
2. After making the 90-second bread, slice and toast it, allow it to cool, and then blitz in a food processor or grate to make breadcrumbs.
3. Heat the oil in a frying pan and add the Pancetta. Cook for 2 - 3 minutes to golden
4. Add the Leek and Celery; cook these over medium / low heat for 3 - 5 minutes to soften but not brown.
5. Remove from heat and allow to cool for a few minutes.
6. Add the Breadcrumbs, Pine nuts, and Thyme to a large mixing bowl. Combine and then add the cooked mix.
7. Add the remaining egg and fully combine.
8. Either transfer the mix into a small lined loaf tin or allow it to cool and stuff Turkey with the mix fully.
9. Bake at 180°C for 30 minutes or until golden if baking as a loaf.

Pizza Casserole

Pork Recipes | **Prep Time:** 10 minutes | **Servings:** 4
Per Serving: Kcal: 607, Carbs (net) 11.7 grams, Fat 42.5 grams, Protein 39.6 grams

Ingredients
- Sandie's Ketchup
- 400g Tinned Tomatoes
- 4 tsp Malt Vinegar
- 2 tsp Truvia / Natvia / Pure Via Sweetener
- 1 tsp Kashmiri Chilli
- 1 tsp Mixed Spice
- Salt & Pepper

Casserole Ingredients
- 600g Cauliflower
- 1 tbsp Italian herbs and spices (reserve a little for the topping)
- 12 Pork Chipolatas (e.g. Aldi 97% pork)
- 100g Courgette
- 100g Leeks, finely sliced (cooked for approx 5 minutes in a little water in the microwave)
- 200g Mozzarella (half for the topping and half to go in the cauliflower base)
- 50g Cheddar
- 60g Cherry Tomatoes

Directions
1. Preheat the oven to 220°C.
2. Cauliflower rice - Chop the cauliflower until it looks like rice/couscous, using your food processor or a strong knife. Chop up the leaves as well!
3. Add to the cauliflower, your Italian seasoning, salt and pepper, 100g mozzarella, and stir
4. Pop this into a greased ovenproof dish

5. Chop up your sausages into small chunks (if using chorizo or pepperoni, miss out on this stage) and scatter evenly across the top of the cauliflower mix
6. Pop in the oven for approx 25 minutes

The Sauce
1. Meanwhile, we'll make the tomato sauce. Put all the sauce ingredients into a bullet or bowl and use a hand blender. Blend till smooth
2. Final Construction
3. Once the cauliflower rice is out of the oven, add your meat (if using ready-cooked meat) and veg toppings. I did shavings of courgette, finely chopped pepper, and leeks.
4. Top with the tomato sauce
5. Scatter your grated mozzarella and grated cheddar
6. Chop your cherry tomatoes in half and even put them on the top.
7. And finally, put a little Italian herbs/spices over the top
8. Oven cook (still 220°c) for about 15 mins, then turn the temperature down to 200°c for a further 15 minutes (total about 30 minutes).

Pork in Pastry Roll

Pork Recipes | **Prep Time:** 20 minutes | **Servings:** 4
Per Serving: Kcal: 365, Carbs (net) 4.2 grams, Protein 32 grams, Fat 22.7 grams

Ingredients
- 1 batch of Suet Pastry (see recipe)
- 475-500g Pork Fillet
- 50g Homemade Tomato Sauce / Sandie's Ketchup / Passata

Directions
1. Follow the instructions for the suet pastry and preheat the oven to 180°C.
2. Between 2 sheets of greaseproof paper, roll out the pastry to a suitable size to wrap the pork fillet.
3. Spread the tomato sauce around the center of the pastry and use greaseproof paper to roll the fillet.
4. Tuck in the ends of the pastry to seal the fillet.
5. Bake for around 10-15 minutes with the greaseproof paper on. The paper should now easily come away from the pastry. Cook for another 35-40 minutes.
6. Once cooked, allow the fillet to rest for 5-10 minutes before slicing.

Pork & Sage Stuffing

Pork Recipes | **Prep Time:** 10 minutes | **Servings:** 8
Per Serving: Kcal: 125, Carbs (net) 1 gram, Protein 9.8 grams, Fat 7.5 grams

Ingredients
- 80-100g breadcrumbs, e.g., one 90 second bread roll, toasted & finely chopped
- 20g Lard or Butter
- 80g White Onion or Shallot, finely chopped
- 2 Garlic Cloves, finely chopped
- 2 tsp Dried Sage or 8-10 Fresh Sage Leaves
- 500g Pork Mince (5%) - or we also use our Ketoroma 97% Pork Sausage Meat!
- 1 Large Egg

Directions
1. Preheat the oven to 180°C.
2. Make the 90-second bread as per the recipe. Slice and toast it until crunchy.
3. Heat the lard or butter gently in a small frying pan.
4. Add the chopped onion and garlic to the pan and soften them without browning for 3-5 minutes. Remove from the heat to cool for a few minutes.
5. In a large mixing bowl, add the pork mince, dried / fresh sage, egg, 90-second bread (crush the bread in your hands to create a mix of large & small breadcrumbs), and the fried onion & garlic.
6. Fully combine these ingredients with your hands and separate them into 12 equal portions.
7. Bake for 20-25 minutes. This can also be made as a stuffing loaf in a small bread tin - cook for an extra 15-20 minutes to ensure the meat is fully cooked.

Pork Schnitzel

Pork Recipes | **Prep Time:** 10 minutes | **Servings:** 2
Per Serving: Kcal: 541, Carbs (net) 3.2 grams, Protein 45.6 grams, Fat 36.1 grams

Ingredients
- 300-350g Pork Fillet
- Salt & Pepper
- 1 tsp Curry Blend
- 30g Coconut Flour
- 1 Egg, beaten
- 70g Cauliflower, grated / 'riced' (use a food processor)
- 30g Ground Almonds / Milled Linseed

- 20g Butter or Cooking Coconut Oil
- 20g Olive Oil

Directions
1. Cover the pork with cling film and bash with a rolling pin to flatten it as much as possible!
2. Cut it in half to make it easier to fry in a pan.
3. Season the pork with salt & pepper.
4. Place the coconut flour in one bowl, the egg in a second bowl, and the cauliflower rice & ground almonds (mixed) in a third bowl.
5. Add half the curry blend to the coconut flour and a half to the egg. Mix thoroughly.
6. Take each piece of pork and place in each mixture: first - coconut flour, second - beaten egg, third - cauliflower & almonds.
7. Heat a pan with the butter and olive oil over medium heat and add the coated pork fillet. Cook them for 3-5 minutes on each side until they're crisp.

Pumpkin Spaghetti Carbonara

Pork Recipes | **Prep Time:** 10 minutes | **Servings:** 4
Per Serving: Kcal: 519, 16.1g Carbs, 30.9g Protein, 37.1g Fat

Ingredients
- 800g Pumpkin - spiralized
- 300g Bacon - diced
- 6 medium eggs
- 60g Parmesan - grated
- 2 garlic cloves, chopped finely
- 20g butter
- 10g Olive oil
- 5g Fresh basil - optional
- Salt and Pepper

Directions
1. Add oil to a large nonstick pan and fry the bacon for approx. 3 - 5 minutes, stirring occasionally
2. Add the butter, spiralized pumpkin, and garlic to the bacon pan and fry until cooked. 5 - 10 minutes
3. In a separate bowl, whisk up the eggs, parmesan, salt, and pepper
4. Once cooked, take the pumpkin off the heat and stir in the egg mix
5. Allow the heat of the pumpkin to cook the egg mix, but don't worry if it ends up scrambling. It'll still taste fabulous
6. Serve immediately, although this does reheat beautifully too

7. Finally, sprinkle some basil and extra parmesan over the top
8. Enjoy :-)

Roast Pepper & Chorizo

Pork Recipes | **Prep Time:** 5 minutes | **Servings:** 4
Per Serving: Kcal: 324, 7g Carbs, 12.5g Protein, 27.8 g Fat

Ingredients
- 500g Mixed Coloured Peppers (weight once prepped)
- 2 tsp Fresh Garlic or 1.5 tsp Garlic Powder
- 200g Chorizo
- 30g Olive Oil
- 1 tsp Salt
- Freshly ground pepper

Directions
1. Preheat oven 190C (Ninja Grill 180C)
2. Chunky chop the peppers & chorizo into a large bowl
3. Add all the other ingredients to the bowl and mix well
4. Pop into an ovenproof dish, and spread out evenly
5. Cook for about 20 - 30 minutes, until cooked
6. Serve hot or cold

Sausage & Leek Mash Pie

Pork Recipes | **Prep Time:** 10 minutes | **Servings:** 2
Per Serving: Kcal: 610, 10.9g Carbs, 40.3g Protein, 43.4g Fat

Ingredients
- 400g Cauliflower Florets
- 4 x 97% Pork Sausages (we use our Ketoroma Pork Sausages)
- 30ml Olive Oil or Coconut oil
- 100g Leek
- 150g Courgette
- A handful of Fresh Parsley, Sage, or Thyme, finely chopped
- 200ml Stock (we use homemade ham stock from page 70, but a stock cube can also be used)
- 1 tsp Garlic Powder
- 15g Butter
- 30g Crème Fraîche
- Salt & Pepper

Directions
1. Preheat the oven to 200°C.

2. Steam the cauliflower florets (we pop them in the microwave, in a covered bowl with a dash of water, for around 4 minutes). It doesn't need to be cooked, just softened to help it break down into a mash.
3. Meanwhile, chop the sausages into bite-sized chunks and roughly chop the courgette and leek. We like to leave these quite chunky.
4. Heat the oil in a pan over gentle heat. Add the leeks, courgette, and parsley to the pan. Allow softening for a few minutes.
5. Add the sausages, combine, cover the pan with a lid and allow the sausages to cook for around 5 minutes.
6. Add the stock, garlic powder, and a dash of salt (we don't use much as our homemade stock contains salt). Cover the pan with a lid to cook through.
7. Add the steamed cauliflower florets to a food processor with the butter. Blitz until it forms your preferred mash consistency
8. Take the lid off the pan, add the crème fraîche and stir through to create a creamy sauce.
9. Transfer the contents of the pan to an oven dish, then top with the cauliflower mash. You could add some grated cheese if you wish :)
10. Bake for around 15 minutes to turn the mash golden.

Sausage Plait

Pork Recipes | **Prep Time:** 20 minutes | **Servings:** 4
Per Serving: Kcal: 429, Carbs (net) 5.6 grams, Protein 24.2 grams, Fat 34.1 grams

Ingredients
- 400g Pork Sausages (97% Pork or above) - we use our Ketoroma Sausage Meat!
- 1 medium (around 150g) Red Pepper, chopped
- 100g Leeks, chopped
- 15ml/g Olive Oil / Butter
- 1/2 tsp Kashmiri Chilli
- 30g Tomato Puree / Sandie's Ketchup
- 1 egg, whisked in a small bowl
- 1 Garlic Clove, finely chopped, or 1/2 tsp Garlic Powder
- Salt & Pepper

Directions
1. Preheat the oven to 180°C.
2. Fry off the leeks and peppers in the olive oil/butter and add some seasoning.
3. Remove the sausage meat from the skin and place the meat into a bowl.

4. Add the chilli, tomato sauce, garlic, seasoning, and half of the whisked egg to the meat.
5. Add the cooked peppers and leeks to the meat and combine.
6. Make your MKD as per the recipe (see here). Work with this while it's still hot.
7. Roll the dough out into a rectangle to the length of your baking tray and then transfer it to a lined baking tray.
8. Place the meat filling in the middle of the dough and spread it out along the middle of the rectangle. Leave a little gap between the meat and the end of the pasty - about 3cm.
9. Cut the dough at a slight diagonal on either side of the filling into about 1.5cm strips. Make the same number of cuts on each side.
10. Tuck the top and bottom edges of the pastry over the filling. Then take each strip and lay it over the meat, alternating between sides.
11. Pop in the oven for approximately 30 minutes. If you have a thermometer, the inside is cooked when it reaches 83°C. It should be golden & crispy :)

Savoy Carbonara

Pork Recipes | **Prep Time:** 20 minutes | **Servings:** 4
Per Serving: Kcal: 585, Carbs (net) 12.1 grams, Protein 34.8 grams, Fat 41.6 grams

Ingredients
- 400g Savoy Cabbage
- 250g Gammon Steak (smoked or unsmoked)
- 50g Shallots
- 20g Butter
- 1/2 tsp Garlic Powder
- 60g Mascarpone Cheese
- 100g Soured Cream
- 20g Parmesan Cheese

Directions
1. Chop the savoy cabbage into strips, dice the gammon steaks, and chop the shallots.
2. Melt the butter in a large pan/wok over medium heat.
3. Fry the gammon steaks, shallots, and garlic powder in the butter and cook over medium heat for 5-6 minutes until the shallots soften and the gammon changes color to a darker shade.

4. Add the shredded savoy cabbage and combine. Cover with a lid and allow to cook for a further 5-8 minutes. The cabbage will turn a deeper shade of green.
5. Add the mascarpone and sour cream and stir well. Re-cover and allow to cook for 2-3 minutes to let the mascarpone create the sauce.
6. Divide into two portions and top with grated parmesan :)

Pork in Rich Tomato Sauce

Pork Recipes | **Prep Time:** 10 minutes | **Servings:** 2
Per Serving: Kcal: 493, Carbs (net) 8.5 grams, Protein 38 grams, Fat 33 grams

Ingredients
- 15g Butter / Olive Oil
- 1-2 Garlic Cloves, chopped
- 100g Carrot, roughly chopped
- 100g Leeks, roughly chopped
- 2 Pork Shanks (or use a joint with crackling)
- 250ml Vegetable Stock (we use Bouillon - this isn't clean keto)
- 10-15 leaves of Fresh Sage or 1 tsp Dried Sage
- 15g Tomato Puree

Directions
1. Start by melting the butter in a pan over medium heat and gently frying the garlic, carrots, and leek for 3-5 minutes.
2. Transfer these into your slow cooker, and add the pork joint/shanks, stock, and sage. Leave the tomato puree out until the end.
3. Slow cook on high for 4 hours or low for 8 hours.
4. Lift the meat from the slow cooker at the end of the slow cooking process. Remove the fat layer and roast this without the meat in a hot oven until crispy (around 30-40 minutes) to create crackling!
5. If you have a stick blender, you can blitz the veg & stock together while hot (be careful!). If you're using a jug blender, wait until it has cooled sufficiently before blending.
6. Add the tomato puree to the sauce and blitz to your preferred consistency. Season to taste.
7. We served the pork on a bed of buttered cabbage :)

Swedish Style Meatballs

Pork Recipes | **Prep Time:** 20 minutes | **Servings:** 4
Per Serving: Kcal: 395, 3.6g Carbs, 43.5g Protein, 22.5g Fat

Ingredients
- 30ml Olive Oil or Coconut Oil
- 100g Shallots, finely chopped
- 1-2 Garlic Cloves, finely chopped
- 80g 'Breadcrumbs' (e.g., one 90 second bread)
- 1/4 tsp Ground Nutmeg or a good grating of Fresh Nutmeg
- 500g Pork Mince (5% Fat)
- 1 Large Egg
- 300ml Beef Stock
- 1-1.5 tsp Dijon Mustard
- 50g Soured Cream
- Salt & Pepper
- Fresh herbs to garnish

Directions
1. Heat 1 tbsp oil in a pan and finely chop the shallot. Add to the pan and cook until soft and translucent.
2. Add the garlic, cook for a further minute, and then leave to cool.
3. Mix the pork mince, breadcrumbs, shallots, egg, nutmeg, and seasoning until combined, then form 16 meatballs. Chill the meatballs for 15 mins in the fridge.
4. Heat the remaining oil in the pan. Add your chilled meatballs and cook for 5 - 10 mins, occasionally turning until browned all over.
5. Add the stock and simmer for around 8-10 mins to reduce slightly.
6. Stir in the mustard and sour cream, season to taste, and serve.

SEAFOOD RECIPES

Baked Basa Fillet

Seafood Recipes | **Prep Time:** 10 minutes | **Servings:** 1
Per Serving: Kcal: 456, Carbs (net) 11 grams, Protein 47.8 grams, Fat 26.1 grams

Ingredients
- 190g Basa Fillet (or Cod or Haddock fillets)
- 50g Leek or Spring Onions, finely sliced
- 50g Red / Yellow Peppers, finely sliced
- 100g Coconut Milk (as high % coconut extract as you can get) - can be swapped with Soured Cream or Greek / Greek-Style Yogurt
- 5ml Lemon Juice
- 1/2 tsp Ground Cumin
- 1 tsp Ground Coriander
- 1/2 tsp Ginger Puree
- 1/8 tsp (a pinch) Cayenne Pepper

Directions
1. Preheat the oven to 180°C.
2. Spread the peppers & leek/spring onions on the bottom of a small oven-proof dish.
3. Lay the fish fillet either in small strips or while fillet over the peppers & onions.
4. Mix the coconut milk, lemon juice, and spices and evenly spread them over the fish.
5. Cover the dish with foil and bake for 25-30 minutes.
6. E straight from the dish or use a spatula to lift from the dish. Don't discard the excess liquid! Serve with a low-carb veggies/salad and dress with the infused liquid.

Chilli & Lime Cod

Seafood Recipes | **Prep Time:** 10 minutes | **Servings:** 2
Per Serving: Kcal: 194, Carbs (net) 2.4 grams, Protein 27.3 grams, Fat 8.8 grams

Ingredients
- 2 Boneless & Skinless Cod Fillets
- 1/2 tsp Paprika
- 10g Fresh Parsley, finely chopped (or 1 tsp Dried Parsley)
- 1/4 tsp Chilli Flakes
- 1/4 tsp Garlic Powder
- 1/4 tsp Ground Cumin
- 15ml Olive Oil
- Zest and juice of 1 small lime

Directions

1. Mix the oil with the spices, herbs, lime zest, and half of the juice - save the rest of the juice as a dressing on the plate.
2. Place the cod fillets in a dish and spoon over the oil & spice mix. Allow this to sit in the fridge for 20-30 minutes minimum (overnight is best).
3. Preheat the oven to 180°C and cook for 15 minutes or fry in a good non-stick frying pan over medium heat for 6-8 minutes. The fillet should be firm when fully cooked.
4. Serve with a fresh salad and drizzle with the remaining lime juice.

Keto Fish Bites

Seafood Recipes | **Prep Time:** 10 minutes | **Servings:** 2
Per Serving: Kcal: 495, 1.5g Carbs, 43.2g Protein, 34.7g Fat

Ingredients
- 375g Fresh Skinless Fish - Macros are for Skinless Cod
- 3 Large Eggs
- Coconut Oil / Lard for frying (500g-1kg, depending on the size of your pan)

Directions
1. Dice the fish and place it into a small food blender.
2. Add the eggs to the blender and any seasoning you choose - Our favourites are Smoked Paprika and Garlic (1/2 tsp of each) / 1 tsp Keto & Spice Curry Blend / 1/2 tsp, Dried Dill
3. Blitz the fish & eggs for 15 - 20 seconds. Don't over blend this - it should look like a lumpy paste.
4. Heat the oil in a large frying pan/wok to 190 degrees - use a thermometer to check the temperature.
5. Add a dessert spoon of the mix to the oil at a time once the oil is full to temperature. Don't add too many as this will reduce the temperature of the oil.
6. Cook for around 5 minutes or until the fish bites are cooked thoroughly - above 63 degrees.
7. Remove the bites from the oil and place absorbent paper to remove any excess oil.

Fresh Pepper Salad with Anchovies

Seafood Recipes | **Prep Time:** 5 minutes | **Servings:** 4
Per Serving: Kcal: 252, 6.1g Carbs, 9.4g Protein, 20.1g Fat

Ingredients
- 500g Peppers - Sliced thinly
- 80g Spring Onions - Sliced thinly
- 2 tsp Freshly garlic, finely chopped
- 30g Olive oil
- 1tsp Salt
- Freshly ground pepper
- 1tsp Paprika
- 80g Roasted Almonds - I fried mine in 20g butter, but you can dry fry them in a non-stick saucepan
- 60g Anchovies - optional, but I have included these in the macros
- 15g Basil leaves

Directions
1. Add your flaked almonds to a pan, dry fry, or add a little butter. Fry until golden brown.
2. Add all your ingredients to a large bowl, including the golden flaked almonds, and mix.

Garlic Prawns

Seafood Recipes | **Prep Time:** 5 minutes | **Servings:** 1
Per Serving: Kcal: 358, Carbs (net) 1.6 grams, Protein 36.2 grams, Fat 23 grams

Ingredients
- 20g Butter or Olive Oil
- 1-2 Garlic Cloves, sliced
- 200g Raw King Prawns
- 20g Fresh Coriander, finely chopped
- Juice of 1/2 a lemon

Directions
1. If using frozen prawns, ensure these are fully defrosted and drained.
2. Melt the butter/oil in a small frying pan over medium heat.
3. Add the garlic and allow to fry gently for 2-3 minutes to begin to turn golden brown.
4. Add the prawns and increase the heat a little. Cover the pan and allow to cook for 2-3 minutes.
5. Remove the lid and turn the prawns to ensure they cook throughout.
6. Add the coriander and squeeze the lemon juice over the prawns. Combine and serve.

Paella (Haddock & Chorizo)

Seafood Recipes | **Prep Time:** 10 minutes | **Servings:** 4
Per Serving: Kcal: 367, 11.4g Carbs, 37.4g Protein, 16.4g Fat

Ingredients
- 30ml Olive Oil
- 100g Shallots, finely sliced
- 3 Garlic Cloves, finely sliced
- 100g Red Bell Pepper, finely sliced
- 60g Chorizo, diced
- 800g Cauliflower
- 200ml Stock (chicken / fish) or water
- 2 tsp Smoked Paprika
- 1 tsp Pink Himalayan / Rock Salt
- 1/2 - 1 tsp Chilli Flakes
- A handful of Fresh Flat Leaf Parsley, finely chopped (save some for topping)
- 200g Passata
- 600g Haddock Fillets (skinless)
- Salt & Pepper

Directions
1. Heat the olive oil in a large pan over low heat.
2. Add the shallots, garlic, pepper, and chorizo. Allow the veg to soften and the oil from the chorizo to seep out.
3. Meanwhile, break the cauliflower into florets and blitz in a food processor until it resembles rice.
4. By this point, the oil in the bottom of the pan should be orange. Add the cauliflower rice and combine with the veg & chorizo.
5. Add the stock/water to the pan, the passata, smoked paprika, salt, chilli flakes, and parsley. Cover the pan with a lid for a few minutes.
6. Remove the lid, give the rice a quick mix, and lay the fish on top (break this into large chunks - some will flake as the dish cooks). Cover the pan with a lid again.
7. After 6 - 8 minutes, remove the lid and carefully combine the fish with the rice. Season to taste and serve.

Keto Kedgeree

Seafood Recipes | **Prep Time:** 10 minutes | **Servings:** 2
Per Serving: Kcal: 448, Carbs (net) 10.5 grams, Protein 43.7 grams, Fat 25.3 grams

Ingredients
- 600g Cauliflower / Broccoli (we save broccoli stalks and use this for the 'rice')
- 40g Butter / Olive Oil
- 250g Smoked Haddock
- 80g Shallots / Leeks

- 2 tsp Ground Turmeric
- 1 tsp Curry Powder (we use our Curry Blend - you don't need the additional turmeric if using this)
- 1/2 tsp Hot Chilli
- 2 Large Eggs (these can either be scrambled into the rice or hardboiled and chopped)

Directions

1. Shred the cauliflower or broccoli into 'rice' with a food processor (or use store-bought riced cauliflower/broccoli).
2. Melt half of the butter/oil in a large frying pan/wok over medium heat and add the fish, skin side down. Place a lid on the pan and cook for 5-8 minutes until the fish flakes are firm.
3. Remove the fish from the pan and place it on a plate to cool.
4. Add the rest of the butter/oil to the pan and heat over medium heat.
5. Dice the shallots/leeks and fry gently for 3-5 minutes until they are soft but not brown.
6. Turn the heat up to maximum and add the cauliflower/broccoli rice. Combine with the shallots/leeks and fry for 1-2 minutes.
7. Reduce the heat to low and cover the pan with a lid to allow the cauliflower/broccoli to cook.
8. Add the spices. You may need to add a couple of tablespoons of water to combine all of the spices fully.
9. There are 2 ways to add the egg to the dish - either crack the eggs directly into the rice and combine, cooking for 1-2 minutes to ensure the egg is fully cooked, or add chopped hardboiled eggs.
10. Add the fish back to the rice (remove the skin if you want), breaking the fillets into bite-sized pieces. Season and serve, adding a spoon of soured cream to finish (optional).

Rice Dish- Fish Paella

Seafood Recipes | **Prep Time:** 20 minutes | **Servings:** 4
Per Serving: Kcal: 380, 17g Carbs, 34.5g Protein, 17g Fat

Ingredients
- Follow the recipe for Rice Base Dish
- 200g Red Pepper - Chunky chopped
- 600g Fish of your choice, or seafood mix - keep it whole as it will naturally flake while being cooked
- 400g Tinned tomatoes
- 3tsp Paprika

- 50g Olives - halved
- 1 Lemon (1/2 to squeeze in the recipe & 1/2 to cut into 4 wedges)
- 25g Fresh parsley
- Salt & Pepper
- 20g Olive oil

Directions

1. Follow the instructions for the Rice Base Dish
2. In a non-stick saucepan, add the tinned tomatoes, olives, paprika, salt and pepper, and fish. Bring to boil and then turn down to a gentle simmer until cooked through. Approx. 15 minutes
3. Meanwhile, add the oil and heat until sizzling in a frying pan, then add the peppers. Fry until completely cooked
4. Once cooked, add all the ingredients, including the fresh parsley, to the Rice Base recipe and stir through
5. This can be quickly stir-fried to reheat the rice dish or popped into the fridge
6. To reheat, either stir fry or microwave. If reheating in the oven, make sure you cover the dish with foil so it doesn't dry out

Prawns & Tomato Courgetti

Seafood Recipes | **Prep Time:** 10 minutes | **Servings:** 2
Per Serving: Kcal: 474, Carbs (net) 11.5 grams, Protein 32.2 grams, Fat 31.9 grams

Ingredients
- 30ml Olive Oil
- 25g Shallots, finely chopped
- 3-4 Garlic Cloves, thinly sliced
- 200g Tinned Chopped Tomatoes
- 1 Dried Red Chilli (optional)
- 100g (10-12) Baby Plum Tomatoes
- 400g Courgetti (we use the outside of the courgette and save the middle for the Leek & No-Potato Zoup!)
- 60g Mascarpone
- 280-300g Raw Headless King Prawns, fresh or frozen
- 30g Grated Parmesan
- Salt & Pepper to taste

Directions

1. Add the olive oil to a medium pan and sauté the shallots over low heat for 5-7 minutes.
2. Turn the heat up a little, create a well in the shallots and sprinkle in the garlic.

3. Cook over low/medium heat to turn the garlic nut brown. As soon as the garlic has turned, add the tinned tomatoes, crush the chilli into the sauce and add a little water or unsweetened almond milk (no more than 100ml).
4. Cook gently for 10 minutes and wait for the oil to rise to the surface. Halfway through, add the baby plum tomatoes.
5. Thinly slice the courgettes into strips.
6. Add the courgette to salted, boiling water and blanch for 3-5 minutes.
7. Once the sauce has thickened, add the mascarpone and stir it in.
8. Drain the courgette.
9. Add the prawns to the sauce and cook for 3-5 minutes over medium heat.
10. Add the courgette to the pan and fully combine with the prawns and sauce.
11. Serve in a pasta bowl with a drizzle of olive oil and shards of parmesan cheese.

Salmon & Broccoli Bake

Seafood Recipes | **Prep Time:** 10 minutes | **Servings:** 2
Per Serving: Kcal: 510, Carbs (net) 4.6 grams, Protein 35 grams, Fat 36 grams

Ingredients
- 300ml/g Unsweetened Almond Milk (or another non-dairy alternative)
- A couple of sprigs of Fresh Dill or 1/2 tsp Dried Dill (or use Chives or Parsley)
- 200g Broccoli Florets
- 2 Salmon Fillets (approx. 120g raw weight each)
- 60g Mascarpone (alternatively, use Soft Cream Cheese or Soured Cream)
- 60g Grated Mozzarella (choose a stronger cheese if you prefer)

Directions
1. Preheat the oven to 180°C.
2. In a small saucepan, heat the milk over medium heat, add the sprigs of dill, and allow to bubble gently (not boil).
3. Add the broccoli florets and allow them to simmer for 3-4 minutes to soften.
4. While the broccoli is simmering, cut the salmon into chunks. If you want to remove the skin, do so before cutting it into chunks.
5. Add the salmon to the broccoli and allow to cook for 2-3 minutes.
6. Stir in the mascarpone to thicken the sauce, season, and then transfer to an ovenproof dish.
7. Scatter the cheese over the top and bake for 10-15 minutes or until golden brown.

Salmon Terrine

Seafood Recipes | **Prep Time:** 20 minutes | **Servings:** 4
Per Serving: Kcal: 342, 2.9g Carbs, 18g Protein, 29g Fat

Ingredients
- 400g Smoked Salmon - if you're making 1 large taurine, you won't need as much. 300g will be more than enough
- 250g Cream Cheese
- 100g Very soft butter, but not liquid. My kitchen was particularly cold, so I gave it a quick blast in the microwave
- 150g Cooked Salmon - flaked into very small pieces
- 100g Cucumber - skinned & finely chopped - These are for the filling
- 120g Cucumber - skinned & very finely sliced - these are for the base
- Whole lemon zest
- 1 tbsp lemon juice, approx half lemon juice
- 2 tsp wholegrain mustard or horseradish - both are delicious
- 2 Tbsp Chives - finely chopped
- Salt & Pepper - season to taste
- 1 Tbsp Dill for decoration
- Some lemon slices to decorate

Directions
- Lightly oil your tin or ramekins with oil (water will work as well) & then line it with clingfilm. Make sure there is plenty of cling film hanging over the outside of your ramekins or tin
- Grind black pepper into the base of the clingfilm-lined tin or ramekins. then place your lemon slices and finally break pieces of dill and place them in the base or bases
- If you're doing individual ramekins, it's 50g of smoked salmon per ramekin. Completely line your dishes/tin with the slices of smoked salmon. Allow the salmon to drape over the outside

The Filling
1. Add to a food processor - Cream Cheese, softened butter, lemon zest & lemon juice & whiz till smooth
2. Transfer to a large bowl
3. Now add all the other ingredients - flaked salmon, 100g finely chopped cucumber, whole grain mustard or horseradish, finely chopped chives
4. Mix well, taste now season with salt & pepper & mix again

5. Compact it well into your dishes, and then put your finely sliced cucumber over the top, completely sealing the filling
6. Fold the remaining lost bits of smoked salmon over the top of the cucumber. If it completely seals the cucumber, great. If not, that's fine too :-)
7. Now seal the dish with the overhanging clingfilm
8. With your hands, gently compact it into the dish/dishes and chill for a couple of hours.
9. So long as all the ingredients are fresh, this will keep in the fridge for a few days
10. To turn out of the dish/dishes, open up the clingfilm, pop a plate on top, and turn it upside down, et voila!

Salmon Wellington

Seafood Recipes | **Prep Time:** 10 minutes | **Servings:** 4
Per Serving: Kcal: 620, Carbs (net) 4.4 grams, Fat 49 grams, Protein 38 grams

Ingredients
- 4 x 120g Salmon Fillets
- 100g Baby Leaf Spinach
- 60g Mascarpone Cheese
- 100g Ground Almonds or Milled Seeds (e.g., milled linseed)
- 50g Butter
- 1 Large Egg
- 20g Coconut Flour
- 25g Grated Parmesan
- 1/4 tsp Xanthan Gum

Directions
1. Firstly make the pastry. Using a small food processor, add the ground almonds, parmesan, and xanthan gum and mix for a couple of seconds.
2. Add 25g of the butter and blitz for a few seconds.
3. Repeat the step with the remaining butter. The mix should now resemble bread crumbs.
4. Add the egg and mix for 15-20 seconds, so the mix starts to form a dough but doesn't overmix.
5. Transfer the mix to another bowl and add the coconut flour. Mix using a spatula or spoon - this will thicken the pastry.
6. If you are making individual portions, separate the dough into 4 equal portions and roll each out between 2 sheets of greaseproof paper to around 15 cm round / 6 inches.

7. Using a frying pan with a well-fitting lid, wilt the spinach over medium / low heat (you may need to add a little water to start the spinach to wilt.
8. Once the spinach has wilted, add the mascarpone cheese, and cook over low heat until the mascarpone is fully combined with the spinach.
9. Allow the spinach to cool a little before making the parcels.
10. Using one piece of pastry, lay a salmon fillet in the center, add a small amount of wilted spinach and evenly spread along the fillet. Sprinkle with any herbs and seasoning before sealing the pastry.
11. Using the greaseproof, bring in the pastry to wrap the fillet. Use the paper to help you press the pastry in place.
12. Transfer the fillets to a baking tray and bake at 180c for 20 - 25 minutes.
13. For a larger fillet, bake for an extra 10 minutes.

Smoked Haddock & Leek Risotto

Seafood Recipes | **Prep Time:** 10 minutes | **Servings:** 2
Per Serving: Kcal: 331, Carbs (net) 11 grams, Protein 35 grams, Fat 15 grams

Ingredients
- 20g Unsalted Butter
- 200g Leek, finely sliced
- 1-2 Garlic Cloves, finely sliced
- 400g Cauliflower Rice (either rice this yourself in a food processor, or buy it pre-riced)
- 5g Vegetable Bouillon dissolved in 100ml hot water
- 360g Smoked Haddock, skinned and cut into large chunks
- 40g Soured Cream
- A couple of sprigs of Fresh Dill (or 1/2 tsp dried dill)
- Salt & Pepper to taste

Directions
1. Heat the butter gently in a large sauté / frying pan with a well-fitting lid.
2. Add the sliced leeks and garlic and cook for 3-5 minutes to soften.
3. Add the cauliflower rice, combine well with the leeks, and cook for 2 minutes.
4. Add the stock and stir through the rice, lay the haddock fillets on the rice, and place the lid on the pan.
5. Keep the heat low/medium to allow the dish to cook gently for 10-12 minutes.
6. Remove the lid and check the fish is cooked - it should be firm.

7. Gently break the fish into the rice mix. If there is excess liquid, just turn the heat to high for a minute to allow it to evaporate.
8. Reduce the heat, add the soured cream and the dill and gently combine.
9. Season to taste.

Smothered Salmon

Seafood Recipes | **Prep Time:** 10 minutes | **Servings:** 3
Per Serving: Kcal: 257, 1.1g Carbs, 31.9g Protein, 13.4g Fat

Ingredients
- 500g Salmon Fillet
- 25g Greek (Greek Style) Yogurt
- 1 tsp (3g) Mustard Seeds
- 1 tsp (3g) Garlic Powder
- 1 - 2 tsp (3 - 6g) Smoked Paprika - adjust to taste
- 1/2 tsp Ground Pink Salt

Directions
1. Crush the mustard seeds in a pestle and mortar, or crush between 2 spoons.
2. In a small bowl or the Pestle and Mortar, combine the yogurt with the spices - crushed mustard seeds, garlic, paprika, and salt.
3. Place the Salmon on a baking tray and smother it with the yogurt paste.
4. If cooking in the Ninja Grill, preheat the grill and place the salmon directly onto the hot grill plate.If cooking in a conventional oven, first sear the skin by heating 10ml coconut oil in a frying pan and place the salmon in the pan for 2 - 3 minutes. While the salmon is in the pan, place the baking tray in the oven to heat
5. Remove the salmon from the pan and place it on the baking sheet.
6. Bake at 200c for 12 - 15 minutes.
7. To ensure the salmon is fully cooked, use a food temperature probe to check the thickest part of the fillet is at a minimum of 45c.
8. Using the Ninja Grill with the probe, the cooking process will end when the fish has reached 45c unless you adjust the required temperature.

Keto Tuna Bake

Seafood Recipes | **Prep Time:** 10 minutes | **Servings:** 2
Per Serving: Kcal: 522, Carbs (net) 11.2 grams, Protein 44.3 grams, Fat 33.8 grams

Ingredients
- 20g Butter / 20ml Olive Oil
- 80g Shallots or Leeks, finely chopped
- 100g Broccoli Florets, chopped
- 100g Red Bell Pepper, diced
- 100g Aubergine or Courgette, diced
- 1 Tin of Tuna in Spring Water (drained weight = approx. 110g)
- 5 Large Eggs
- 60g Cheddar Cheese, grated (or other cheese of choice

Directions
1. Preheat the oven to 180°C.
2. Add the butter/oil to a medium saucepan and fry the diced shallots/leeks, broccoli, pepper, and aubergine/courgette for 3-5 minutes over medium heat until the veg starts to soften but not brown.
3. Add the drained can of tuna and combine this with the veg. Cook for a further 2-3 minutes.
4. Transfer the mix into an oven-proof dish (or two smaller dishes).
5. Beat the eggs in a bowl with a pinch of salt and pour this over the tuna & veg. Sprinkle the grated cheese on top.
6. Bake for 35-45 minutes or until the mix is firm and golden brown.

Tuna & Broccoli Fishcakes

Seafood Recipes | **Prep Time:** 10 minutes | **Servings:** 2
Per Serving: Kcal: 290, Carbs (net) 3.4 grams, Protein 27.5 grams, Fat 17.4 grams

Ingredients
- 1 Tin (112g drained weight) Tuna in Spring Water
- 100g Broccoli Florets, cooked & cooled
- 40g Ground Almonds / Milled Linseed
- 10g Psyllium Husks
- 2 Large Eggs, beaten
- Season & spice to taste - garlic/onion powder would work nicely

Directions
1. Preheat the oven to 180°C if baking the fishcakes.
2. Mix all ingredients in a large mixing bowl and rest for 5 mins (this allows the psyllium to bind the mix).
3. Divide the mix into 4.
4. To pan-fry, use an egg ring to help form the fish cake, pressing it into shape. Fry for 5 minutes over low-medium heat with the egg ring in place. Remove the ring and turn the fish cake to cook on both sides.

5. To oven bake, shape the fish cakes by hand, place them on a baking sheet, or use a small non-stick baking tin. Bake for 25-30 minutes until firm.

Turmeric Basa Fillet

Seafood Recipes | **Prep Time:** 10 minutes | **Servings:** 2
Per Serving: Kcal: 253, Carbs (net) 2.6 grams, Protein 33 grams, Fat 12.6 grams

Ingredients
- 380g Basa Fillets - Defrosted and drained
- 20ml Olive Oil
- 1/2 Tsp Ground Turmeric
- 2 Garlic Cloves / 5 g Garlic Puree
- 1/2 inch Fresh Ginger Root / 5 g Ginger Puree
- 20 g Fresh Coriander / Small handful chopped
- Salt to season

Directions
1. Use either a pestle and mortar or a small blender/grinder to mix the oil, turmeric, ginger, garlic, and coriander to create a paste.
2. Ensure you have defrosted the fish and drained away any moisture.
3. Put the fillets on a plate or small tray and spoon the paste on the fish using the back of the spoon to coat all the fish. Turn the fillets to coat both sides.
4. Allow the fish to rest for a few minutes (these can be prepped the night before and stored in the fridge,
5. Heat a good non-stick pan over medium heat. Once hot, add the fish fillets and cook for 4 - 5 minutes.
6. Carefully turn the fillets and cook for a further 3 - 4 minutes.

TURKEY RECIPES

Sandie's Pimped Up Christmas Turkey

Turkey Recipes | **Prep Time:** 10 minutes | **Servings:** 6
Per Serving: Kcal: 714, 9.3g Carbs, 71.2g Protein, 42.5g Fat

Ingredients
- A Turkey (obviously)
- 125g Butter, softened
- 30ml Olive Oil
- 2 tsp Ketoroma Poultry Blend (alternatively, use 2 crushed cloves of garlic and 1/4 tsp ground turmeric)
- 2 tsp Smoked Paprika
- Salt to taste
- Freshly Ground Black Pepper
- 1 Medium Orange, studded with 9 Cloves
- A handful of Fresh Thyme
- 3 Carrots
- 3 Celery Sticks
- 3 Shallots, chopped in half (leave the skin on)

Directions
1. Mix the butter, olive oil, poultry blend, smoked paprika, salt, and black pepper in a bowl.
2. Place the orange and the thyme in the bird's cavity and then spread the spiced butter mixture all over the blend.
3. Place some butter under the skin of the breast to add more flavour.
4. Gently create an opening between the skin and the meat. Without tearing the skin, place the butter in and massage.
5. Place the turkey in a deep oven tray on top of the whole carrots, celery, and shallots, and then gently pour boiling water into the dish - about an inch deep. This will act as a steamer, keeping the turkey moist.
6. Cover with foil and follow the cooking instructions for the turkey, basting constantly.
7. Remove the foil 20 minutes before the turkey has finished cooking, turn up the heat a little, and brown the skin, continuing to baste the turkey. Take approx. 120ml of the basting fat out and set aside.
8. To give the turkey the ultimate finish, place it on a warmed Christmas platter, decorate with holly leaves and a few frozen cranberries between where the legs are tied - slightly open them, allowing the berries to rest on top without falling off comfortably.

9. Take the basting fat that we set aside and glaze the whole bird, giving a wonderful glow to your centerpiece.

Turkey Bolognese

Turkey Recipe | **Prep Time:** 10 minutes | **Servings:** 4
Per Serving: Kcal: 275, Carbs (net) 6 grams, Protein 41 grams, Fat 9 grams

Ingredients
- 30 ml Olive Oil / Butter / Coconut Oil
- 500g Turkey Mince (2% Fat)
- 100g Leeks, finely chopped
- 200g Sliced Mushrooms
- 1 tsp Dried Mixed Herbs
- 2 Garlic Cloves (chopped) or 1 tsp Garlic Powder
- 400 gm (1 tin) Chopped Tomatoes
- Optional: for a creamy sauce, add 100g mascarpone / soured cream

Directions
1. Heat the oil/butter over medium heat and gently fry the leek and garlic for around 3-5 minutes.
2. Turn the heat up a little, add the mushrooms and fry for 3-5 minutes.
3. Either remove the mushrooms & leeks from the pan or move to one side.
4. Add the turkey mince and break the meat into small pieces using a spatula.
5. Cook the turkey to ensure all the meat turns from pink to white, and then combine with the mushrooms & leeks.
6. Add the chopped tomatoes, herbs, and seasoning with the heat on high. Bring to boil, cover the pan with a lid and reduce heat to low.
7. Allow cooking for 15-20 minutes on low heat covered.
8. Remove the lid and turn the heat up to medium/high to reduce the sauce. Cook for 5-10 minutes.
9. Add mascarpone / soured cream for a creamy sauce.

Turkey Meatballs & Herby Gravy

Turkey Recipe | **Prep Time:** 10 minutes | **Servings:** 4
Per Serving: Kcal: 316, Carbs (net) 3 grams, Protein 37 grams, Fat 17 grams

Ingredients
- 50g 'Breadcrumbs' - we toast & blitz a 90 Second Roll or some slices of Linseed Bread.
- 50g Shallots, roughly chopped
- 3 Garlic Cloves, crushed

- 25g Parmesan, grated (plus more for serving)
- 1 tsp Dried Parsley (or a handful of fresh parsley leaves, chopped)
- 1 tsp Dried Sage (or a handful of fresh sage leaves, chopped)
- 500g Turkey Mince (we used 2% Fat)
- 15g Fresh Soured Cream or Greek / Greek-Style Yogurt
- 20g Cooking Coconut Oil (this is unflavoured) or Olive Oil
- 5g Vegetable Bouillon / Stock Cube mixed with 250ml Hot Water
- 30g Mascarpone Cheese
- Salt & Pepper

Directions
1. Using a food processor, blitz the bread into crumbs. Add the shallots, garlic, parmesan, and herbs - blitz again for 20-30 seconds.
2. Gradually add the meat while the processor is on low to combine with the seasoning mix. Once all the meat has been added, mix in the soured cream, and you should now have a fairly smooth paste.
3. Divide the mix into 12-16 meatballs.
4. Heat the oil in a frying pan (or a large pan that you can cover with a lid) over medium heat and add the meatballs. Gently fry them, letting them brown on all sides for 2-3 minutes.
5. Turn the heat down to low and add half of the stock to the pan. Cover and allow the meatballs to gently cook for 8-10 minutes.
6. Once cooked, place the meatballs in a serving dish to keep them warm.
7. Add the remaining stock to the pan and bring to boil. Add the mascarpone cheese and stir to create a creamy gravy.
8. Pour the gravy over the meatballs and sprinkle with a little parsley & parmesan. We serve this with buttered cabbage and salad :)

Turkey & Bacon Meatloaf

Turkey Recipe | **Prep Time:** 10 minutes | **Servings:** 4
Per Serving: Kcal: 377, Carbs (net) 2.3 grams, Protein 42.9 grams, Fat 23.3 grams

Ingredients
- 40g Butter or 40ml Olive Oil / Coconut Oil
- 200g Courgette, diced
- 100g Leeks, finely chopped
- 8 Rashers of Streaky Bacon

- 500g Turkey Mince (we use 7% fat)
- 1 tsp Dried Sage / 8 Sage Leaves, finely chopped
- 1 Large Egg

Directions
1. Preheat the oven to 180°C.
2. Melt the butter/oil in a large frying pan and add the diced vegetables over medium heat. Cook these until golden brown and softened.
3. Set the pan aside to cool for 10-15 minutes.
4. On a sheet of foil, lay 8 slices of streaky bacon side by side and place in a loaf tin.
5. Mix the turkey mince, sage, and egg thoroughly and season in a mixing bowl.
6. Once the vegetables have cooled, combine them with the meat mix and transfer them to the bacon-lined loaf tin.
7. Fold over the ends of the bacon and foil over the top of the meatloaf and bake for 50-60 minutes.
8. To brown the bacon, transfer the meatloaf from the loaf tin onto a roasting tray and pop it back in the oven for 15-20 minutes.

Turkey & Mozzarella Burgers

Turkey Recipe | **Prep Time:** 10 minutes | **Servings:** 6
Per Serving: Kcal: 127, Carbs (net) 1 gram, Protein 22 grams, Fat 3.5 grams

Ingredients
- 500g Turkey Mince (we use 2% fat)
- 200g Courgette, grated
- 125g Mozzarella Ball
- 20g Tomato Puree
- 1 tsp Dried Basil or a small bunch of Fresh Basil
- 1/2 tsp Pink Himalayan / Rock / Sea Salt
- Optional: 1 tsp Garlic or Onion Powder

Directions
1. Add the turkey mince and grate the courgette into a large mixing bowl.
2. Break the mozzarella (drained of water) into chunks into the processor bowl, and add the fresh herbs, tomato puree, seasoning, and blitz into a lumpy paste.
3. Add the pasta to the mince & courgette and mix well by hand.
4. Separate into 8 equal portions (around 100g each) and pan fry in a good non-stick pan for 8-10 minutes until fully cooked.

Turkey & Serrano Ham Swirl

Turkey Recipe | **Prep Time:** 10 minutes | **Servings:** 2
Per Serving: Kcal: 253, 1.6g Carbs, 37.8g Protein, 10.8g Fat

Ingredients
- 3 slices of Serrano Ham (around 50g)
- 50g Soft Cream Cheese (alternatively, use mascarpone)
- Pinch of herbs
- Pinch of salt
- 1/4 tsp Garlic Powder
- 2 Turkey Steaks (around 240g)

Directions
1. Preheat the oven to 200°C.
2. Lay the slices of Serrano ham on a board so the longer sides of the slices overlap each other slightly.
3. Mix the cream cheese with herbs, salt, garlic powder, and other seasonings in a small bowl.
4. Using the back of a spoon, carefully spread the cream cheese onto the Serrano ham.
5. Lay the turkey steaks between two pieces of cling film and flatten them out slightly using a rolling pin or meat tenderizer.
6. Now lay the turkey steaks on top of the cream cheese. Begin rolling the turkey steaks up by lifting the Serrano ham off the board. See the photos above, which show the direction we roll the turkey steaks in.
7. Place the roll on an oven tray and bake for 20-25 minutes until the turkey is fully cooked. If you slice it through, the meat should be white.

Turkey Slaw

Turkey Recipe | **Prep Time:** 10 minutes | **Servings:** 2
Per Serving: Kcal: 491, Carbs (net) 9 grams, Protein 48.8 grams, Fat 28 grams

Ingredients
- 375g Turkey Steaks - you could use Mini Chicken Fillets instead
- 200g White Cabbage, finely sliced
- 50g Carrot, grated
- 50g Leeks / Shallots, finely sliced
- 50g Mayonnaise (homemade or shop-bought)
- 50g Fresh Soured Cream of Greek Yogurt
- Your choice of seasoning

Directions

1. Suppose using raw Turkey Steaks / Chicken Fillets, pan-fries these in a little olive oil/coconut oil over medium heat. They will take 3-4 minutes on either side. Keep the heat fairly low to prevent them from drying out. While they are cooking, you can prep the coleslaw.
2. Mix the cabbage, carrot, and leek/shallots in a large bowl. Add the mayo and sour cream.
3. Add your choice of seasoning - I'm a massive fan of fresh coriander and chilli, but this dish works with so many different flavours. Smoked paprika and garlic are another household favourite.
4. Once the turkey is fully cooked, allow to cool for a few minutes, and either chop or break into bite-sized pieces and mix with the coleslaw.

Turkey Steaks with a Parmesan Crust

Turkey Recipe | **Prep Time:** 10 minutes | **Servings:** 2
Per Serving: Kcal: 280, Carbs (net) 1 gram, Protein 37 grams, Fat 14 grams

Ingredients
- 240g Turkey Steaks
- 1 Egg
- 25g Ground Almonds or Milled Linseed
- 25g Grated Parmesan
- 1/4 tsp Garlic Powder
- 1/2 tsp Pink Himalayan / Rock / Sea Salt
- 1/2 tsp Dried Parsley

Directions
1. Beat the eggs in a tray/bowl large enough to lay the turkey steaks in.
2. Mix the dry ingredients in a separate bowl.
3. Dip the turkey into the egg on both sides (use forks rather than hands - you'll find it a much cleaner process).
4. Allow any egg to drip off the turkey and add to the bowl with the dry ingredients.
5. Carefully shake the bowl and rotate the steak to cover both sides.
6. Pan-fry the steaks in a good non-stick pan over medium heat for 10-12 minutes, turning 2 or 3 times to ensure the coating goes crispy. Alternatively, place the steaks on the lower wire rack of your air fryer / Ninja Foodi and bake at 200°C for 10-12 minutes.
7. Serve with a fresh green salad or a selection of fresh vegetables.

LAMB RECIPES

Cawl (Lamb Broth)

Lamb Recipe | **Prep Time:** 10 minutes | **Servings:** 4
Per Serving: Kcal: 693, 8.6g Carbs, 56.3g Protein, 46.2g Fat

Ingredients
- 1kg Lamb chunks or lamb mince (I used half of each)
- 250g Leeks - chopped into rough chunks
- 250g Swede - chopped into rough chunks
- 250g Celery - chopped into rough chunks
- 250g Mushrooms - halved
- 100g Celeriac - chopped into rough chunks
- 2 tsp Garlic paste or 1tsp garlic powder or 3 garlic cloves chopped finely
- 1.5 liters of boiling water, with 3 stock cubes
- 50g Parsley - roughly chopped
- Salt & Pepper - I season with 1/2 tsp salt & a generous amount of freshly ground pepper

Optional extra
- A sprinkling of Caerphilly Cheese

Directions
1. Put all the ingredients into a large saucepan APART from the Parsley and mushrooms - I like to add the mushrooms for the last half hour of cooking time, as I like a little bite to the mushrooms - your choice :-)
2. Bring to boil for about 15 minutes and then turn down to a medium to a low simmer for about 2 - 3 hours
3. Cook until all the vegetables and meat are lovely and tender
4. Ladle into 4 deep bowls and sprinkle with parsley

Coriander Kebabs

Lamb Recipe | **Prep Time:** 10 minutes | **Servings:** 4
Per Serving: Kcal: 315, Carbs (net) 1.9 grams, Protein 21.6 grams, Fat 24.8 grams

Ingredients
- 500g Lamb Mince (we use 20% fat)
- 20g Ginger, crushed
- 20g Garlic, crushed
- 20g Coriander, finely chopped
- 20g Fresh Green Chilli, crushed
- 1 tsp Garam Masala
- 1 tsp Pink Himalayan / Rock / Sea Salt

Directions

1. Mix all of the ingredients in a bowl - to allow the spices and herbs to combine properly, spread the meat out around the sides of the bowl and add everything else in the middle, as seen in the photo above.
2. Knead with your hands thoroughly for around 5 minutes.
3. Using wet hands, shape the mince into 12 x 50g balls, then shape each into 10cm long sausages.
4. These can be kept in the fridge or cooked straight away on a griddle pan, in the oven, or grilled on high heat or a BBQ. Each kebab will only take around 10 mins to cook - try to make it crispy on the outside and juicy on the inside.

Doner Kebab

Lamb Recipe | **Prep Time:** 10 minutes | **Servings:** 4
Per Serving: Kcal: 312m, 1.1g Carbs, 21.2g Protein, 24.9g Fat

Ingredients
- 500g Lamb Mince
- 1.5 tsp Cayenne Peper
- 1.5 tsp Garlic Powder
- 1 tsp Pepper
- 1 tsp Mixed Herbs
- 1 tsp Oregano
- 1 tsp Salt
- For an extra kick:
- 1 tsp Kashmiri Chilli
- 1 tsp Chilli Flakes

Directions

1. Place all your herbs and seasoning into a pestle & mortar and pound well.
2. Place your mince into the bowl and add the spice and seasoning mix.
3. Place all of the ingredients into a food processor and blitz well. Alternatively, mix thoroughly with your hands until all the ingredients are combined well. I found a kneading action like you would bread for a few minutes gave the mix a good smooth consistency.
4. Shape your meat into the shape you want and make sure it's pressed as tightly together as possible to form a sliceable block. I used a disposable foil loaf tin and pressed it into that.
5. Place directly into the bottom of your slow cooker and cook for 3-4 hours on high or 7 hours on low, or cover in foil and bake for 45 minutes at 180c in the oven or 170c in the Ninja Foodi.

6. Rest for around 10 minutes before slicing as thin as possible using a vegetable peeler, and enjoy!

Figgis in a Rich Leek Gravy

Lamb Recipe | **Prep Time:** 10 minutes | **Servings:** 4
Per Serving: Kcal: 425, 5.3g Carbs, 30g Protein, 32g Fat

Ingredients
- 20g Butter *
- 100g Leeks - Very finely chopped
- 500g Mince lamb
- 250g Lamb livers - Finely chopped
- 100g Ground Linseed
- 60g Suet
- 1tsp freshly ground pepper
- 1tsp Mixed Spice
- 1tsp Dried thyme or Mixed herbs
- 1tsp Salt
- 2 Beef/lamb stock cubes

The Gravy
- 20g Butter
- 100g Leeks - thinly sliced
- 1.5 Beef/lamb Stock cube
- 600ml Water
- 15g Arrowroot & a little cold water for mixing

Directions

1. In a large pan, melt the butter, add very finely chopped leeks and fry off until cooked but not browned. Approx 5 minutes
2. Meanwhile, add all the other ingredients APART from the suet to a large bowl and mix well
3. Add to the hot pan and fry off until cooked, NOT browned, but NO pink meat - approx 5 minutes
4. If you're making picture No2, this is super quick now; just add the suet, mix through and cook until all the meat is cooked & then move straight on to making the gravy - remove the meat from the pan and then use the same pan, it'll add great flavour to the gravy
5. Back to Picture 1. Allow cooling while you prepare the ramekins
6. You need enough greaseproof paper to line the ramekin, hold the mixture and tie some string around the top - please refer to the picture.
7. Now mix the suet through the cooked meat mixture & stir through well
8. Fill each ramekin equally & pat in gently, like a sandcastle

9. Scrunch the residue greaseproof paper together & twist a bit. Tie some string at the base of this paper - please refer to the picture
10. Cover with a piece of greaseproof paper. Put an elastic band to hold this in place. Tie around the edge of this paper with string to secure it. Take this elastic band off now and repeat on each ramekin - please refer to the picture
11. Place the ramekins into a large lidded saucepan and fill the pan half to two-thirds of the way up the ramekins with boiling water
12. Put a damp tea towel over the top, completely covering all the ramekins. It's ok if the towel drapes into the water - this keeps control of the bubbles
13. Cover with the lid, bring to a boil, and simmer gently for one hour
14. Keep an eye on the water so that it doesn't boil dry and that it doesn't bubble over the height of the bowl, either
15. I set 1 alarm for 60 minutes and another alarm for every 15 minutes to check the water level
16. Once cooked, you can leave them to cool in the pan, or pull them out of the pan and allow them to rest for 5 minutes before turning out onto a plate and gently peeling off the greaseproof paper
17. This pudding heats up well in the microwave for about 20 - 30 seconds

The Gravy
1. Remove the meat from the pan and use this pan to make the gravy. It'll add great flavour. Melt the butter, add the sliced leeks and fry off until cooked but not browned. Approx 5 minutes
2. Add to the pan water & stock cubes & bring to boil
3. Once boiling, in a separate cup, add the arrowroot & add enough water so you can mix it into a runny paste
4. Quickly stir into the stock, keep stirring until the gravy is thick and glossy *
5. Note to the chef - We all like our dressing in different thicknesses. If this isn't thick enough for you, mix a little Arrowroot with water & repeat. Bear in mind that the carbs of arrowroot are 84.75 / 100g. So for the 15g of arrowroot in this recipe, that's 2.1 carbs per portion of gravy
6. I served mine with cauliflower & swede mash. Enjoy :-)

Greek Style Lamb Chops

Lamb Recipe | **Prep Time:** 10 minutes | **Servings:** 3
Per Serving: Kcal: 269, 0.6g Carbs, 14g Protein, 23.3g Fat

Ingredients
- 6 Lamb Chops
- 2 tbsp (30ml) Olive Oil
- Juice of 1 Lemon
- 1 tsp Dried Oregano
- 1 tsp Dried Thyme
- Salt - to taste
- Cracked Black Pepper - to taste

Directions
1. Add the oil, lemon juice, and herbs to a pestle & mortar and mix.
2. Pour this marinade over the lamb and leave it in the fridge covered for at least 1 hour.
3. Remove from the fridge and allow the lamb to come to room temperature.
4. Cook on a hot pan or BBQ (no oil required) for 2 - 3 minutes on each side.
5. Once cooked to your preference, allow resting for 5 minutes before serving.

Italian Inspired Meatballs

Lamb Recipe | **Prep Time:** 10 minutes | **Servings:** 4
Per Serving: Kcal: 363, Carbs (net) 1.4 grams, Protein 23.2 grams, Fat 27.5 grams

Ingredients
- 500g Lamb Mince (other mince can be used)
- 1 Medium Shallot, finely chopped
- Salt & Cracked Black Pepper
- 3-4 Large Garlic Cloves, crushed to a pulp
- A Sprig of Fresh Rosemary, finely chopped
- A Sprig of Fresh Sage, finely chopped
- A Sprig of Fresh Flat Leaf Parsley, finely chopped
- Optional: 10g Black Olives, roughly chopped

Directions
1. First, place all the ingredients in a bowl in the order as it is written in the ingredients list. When you place the meat in the bowl, spread the meat out as much as possible, allowing the ingredients to mix through properly.
2. Once all the ingredients have been added, knead the meat mixture for five minutes.

3. Roll the meat into meatballs (roughly 1-inch diameter) and cook in a pan (no oil is necessary here as the lamb will be fatty enough), under a grill on medium heat, or in an oven for 20 minutes at 200°C.
4. Once cooked, serve with anything you fancy, but we recommend the Tomato & Basil Sauce.
5. Place the meatballs in the sauce and cook for a further 15 minutes to allow the meatballs to stew a little

Kashmiri Chilli & Cinnamon Kofta

Lamb Recipe | **Prep Time:** 10 minutes | **Servings:** 4
Per Serving: Kcal: 340, Carbs (net) 2.6 grams, Protein 22.4 grams, Fat 26.6 grams

Ingredients
- 500g Minced Lamb (we used 20% fat)
- 15g Fresh Ginger, roughly chopped
- 2 Garlic Cloves
- 3 tsp Kashmiri Chilli
- 1 tsp Ground Cinnamon
- A handful of fresh mint
- A handful of fresh coriander
- Salt & Pepper to season
- 15ml Olive Oil

Directions
1. These are best made in a food processor. Place all the ingredients except the olive oil in the processor and blitz to a thick paste. Finely chop the garlic, ginger, and herbs together without a processor, and then mix by hand in a large bowl with the lamb mince.
2. Divide the mix into 4 equal portions and create 3 or 4 koftas from each portion.
3. Heat the oil in a large frying pan over medium heat and add the koftas.
4. Cook for around 10 minutes, rotating them regularly.

Keto Lamb Keema

Lamb Recipe | **Prep Time:** 15 minutes | **Servings:** 4
Per Serving: Kcal: 402, Carbs (net) 6.1 grams, Protein 31.7 grams, Fat 27.8 grams

Ingredients
- 80g Shallots
- 4 Garlic Cloves or 2 tsp Garlic Puree
- 1-inch cube of Ginger or 2 tsp Ginger Puree
- 30ml Olive Oil
- 400g Lamb Mince (10% fat)
- 200g Tinned Chopped Tomatoes

- 2 tsp Ground Turmeric
- 1-2 tsp Garam Masala
- 1/2 - 1 tsp Chilli Flakes
- 100g Paneer Cheese
- 80g Greek or Greek-Style Yogurt
- A handful of chopped coriander

Directions
1. Finely chop the onion, garlic, and ginger, or place them in a food processor and blitz to your preferred consistency.
2. Heat the olive oil in a large saucepan over medium heat and add the shallots, garlic, and ginger mix. Cook gently to soften and brown a little.
3. Add the lamb mince to the onion/garlic mix, breaking the meat apart to aid in cooking the meat thoroughly.
4. Once all of the meat is brown, add the chopped tomatoes and stir. Cover the saucepan and cook on medium heat for 5 minutes.
5. Add the turmeric, garam masala, and chilli flakes and cook over low heat for a few minutes. Check the seasoning. Add salt, pepper, and more chilli if required.
6. Chop the paneer cheese into cubes and add to the dish. Allow it to simmer over low heat for 15-20 minutes.
7. Once you're ready to serve, stir in the yogurt. Serve over salad or cauliflower rice and sprinkle with coriander.

Lamb Ragout

Lamb Recipe | **Prep Time:** 10 minutes | **Servings:** 4
Per Serving: Kcal: 443, Carbs (net) 11.4 grams, Protein 31.6 grams, Fat 29.1 grams

Ingredients
- 600g Diced Lamb Leg
- 60g Butter / Cooking Coconut Oil
- 100g Shallots, chopped
- 100g Carrot, chopped
- 100g Celery, chopped
- 100g Leek, chopped
- 200g Swede, chopped & parboiled in salted water
- 2 Large Garlic Cloves, finely chopped
- 1 tbsp Tomato Puree
- 400g Tinned Chopped Tomatoes
- 400ml Good Quality Stock (see notes above)
- 2 Bay Leaves
- A handful of Fresh Parsley
- Salt & Pepper

Directions

1. Fry off the lamb pieces in the butter over medium/high heat.
2. Once brown, remove the lamb from the pan but leave the fat.
3. Add the shallots, carrot, celery, leek, and swede. Cook the veg until soft but not brown, and you may want to turn the heat down.
4. Add the garlic and tomato puree and stir.
5. Add the lamb pieces, stir, and add the tinned tomatoes & stock. Stir gently, bring to boil, then let it simmer.
6. Add the bay leaves and parsley with the stalks - hold a little back for garnish.
7. Season generously with salt & pepper.
8. Cook for 45-60 minutes very gently, and the sauce will naturally thicken.
9. Remove the bay leaves and parsley and serve.

Lamb Samosa Filling

Lamb Recipe | **Prep Time:** 5 minutes | **Servings:** 16
Per Serving: Kcal: 86, Carbs (net) 1.8 grams, Protein 5.4 grams, Fat 5.9 grams

Ingredients
- 500g Lamb Mince
- 25g Ginger, crushed
- 10g Cloves, crushed
- 1 tsp Garam Masala
- Juice & Zest of 1 Lemon
- 200g Courgette, diced
- 200g Swede, diced and parboiled
- 100g Frozen Peas
- Salt to taste
- A handful of fresh coriander

Directions

1. Place the lamb mince directly into the pan with no oil.
2. Begin to cook, gently releasing the fat from the lamb.
3. Do not brown the lamb - once the fat has rendered and the meat has changed color, add the crushed ginger.
4. Cook for 5 minutes, and add the crushed cloves, garam masala, lemon juice, and zest.
5. Add the courgette and cook the mixture for 10 minutes, constantly turning to prevent the bottom of the pan from burning.
6. Add the swede and the frozen peas and cook for 5 minutes.
7. Season with lots of salt, and don't let the peas over-cook. Let them soften, allowing them to stay green.

8. Take off the heat and let it cool for 10 minutes. Chop the coriander and stir this in.
9. Head to the Samosa Pastry to complete your samosas.

Lamb Shanks in Pesto

Lamb Recipe | **Prep Time:** 10 minutes | **Servings:** 2
Per Serving: Kcal: 392, Carbs (net) 0.7 grams, Protein 31 grams, Fat 29.3 grams

Ingredients
Pesto

- 25ml Olive Oil
- 1-2 Garlic Cloves
- 15g Pine Nuts
- 5g Fresh Basil Leaves (swap these for mint leaves to create a mint pesto)

Plus 2 Lamb Shanks (alternatively, use lamb steaks)

Directions
Pesto

1. This one's super simple... add all of the ingredients into a small food processor/blender and blitz to your preferred texture.

Lamb Shanks

1. Place the lamb shanks in a zip-seal food bag and add the pesto. Massage into the lamb and leave it in the fridge overnight.
2. Preheat the oven to 170°C, wrap each shank in foil and bake on a tray for 90 minutes.
3. Remove the foil and continue to cook for 30-60 minutes - be careful when opening the foil!

Lamb Steak with Middle Eastern Rub

Lamb Recipe | **Prep Time:** 5 minutes | **Servings:** 2
Per Serving: Kcal: 409, Carbs (net) 1 gram, Protein 29 grams, Fat 32 grams

Ingredients
- 300g Lamb Leg Steaks
- 30ml Olive Oil
- 1/4 tsp Dried Coriander
- 1/4 tsp Ground Black Pepper
- 1/4 tsp Ground Cumin
- 1/4 tsp Ground Cinnamon
- 1/4 tsp Hot Chilli
- 1/4 tsp Ground Cloves
- 1/4 tsp Ground Nutmeg
- 1/4 tsp Ground Cardamom
- 1 clove of garlic, finely chopped

- A handful of fresh coriander, roughly chopped

Directions

1. Mix the oil, spices, garlic, and coriander in a small bowl.
2. Rub the mixture over the lamb steaks and leave in the fridge to marinate for at least 2 hours or overnight
3. Heat the oil over medium heat and fry the lamb steaks for 2-3 minutes on each side.
4. Leave to rest for 10 minutes, and then sprinkle with more coriander.
5. Serve with a fresh green salad or a selection of fresh vegetables.

Keto Moussaka

Lamb Recipe | **Prep Time:** 10 minutes | **Servings:** 4
Per Serving: Kcal: 640, Carbs (net) 13.8 grams, Protein 27 grams, Fat 52.7 grams

Ingredients

- 30ml Olive Oil
- 100g Shallots, finely chopped
- 2 Garlic Cloves, crushed
- 500g Lamb Mince
- 1 tsp Ground Cinnamon
- 1 tsp Ground Cumin
- 1 tsp Paprika
- 1/2 tsp Oregano
- 400g (1 tin) Tinned Chopped Tomatoes
- 300g Aubergines, cut into 0.5cm thick slices
- 300g Crème Fraîche
- 100g Cheddar Cheese
- 200g Swede, cut into 0.5cm thick slices and parboiled

Directions

1. Fry off the shallots and garlic in 15ml olive oil until soft, and then add in the lamb mince.
2. Add the cinnamon, cumin, paprika, and oregano once the meat is no longer pink.
3. Cook for 2 minutes and then add the tinned tomatoes and swill out the tin with water. Now cover and gently cook for 30-40 minutes.
4. Season with salt and pepper to taste when the oil comes to the surface.
5. Fry the aubergine slices with 15ml olive oil in a non-stick pan. As each slice is tender (but not too brown), remove them from the pan.

6. Mix the crème fraîche and cheddar in a bowl until thick. Season with salt & pepper.
7. Preheat the oven to 170°C.
8. Assemble the moussaka in a lasagne-style dish. Layer the parboiled swede first and the cooked aubergines, and then add a layer of meat and repeat the process as many times as possible until all the veg and meat mix is used up.
9. Evenly spread the cheese mixture on top.
10. Bake in the oven for approximately 30 minutes.

Moroccan Lamb Steaks

Lamb Recipe | **Prep Time:** 8 minutes | **Servings:** 4
Per Serving: Kcal: 356, Carbs (net) 3 grams, Protein 29 grams, Fat 25 grams

Ingredients

- 600g Lamb Steaks
- 30ml Olive Oil
- Juice of 1 Lemon (around 30ml)
- 3-4 Garlic Cloves, crushed, or 10g Garlic Puree
- 1/4 tsp Hot Chilli Powder
- 1/4 tsp Ground Black Pepper
- 1/2 tsp Ground Pink Himalayan / Rock / Sea Salt
- 1 tsp Dried Mint (or a small bunch of fresh mint, finely chopped)
- 1 tsp Smoked Paprika
- 1 tsp Ground Cumin
- 1 tbsp Ground Coriander
- Extra Fresh Mint for garnish

Directions

1. Mix all the ingredients except the lamb and the extra mint to create a paste in a small bowl.
2. Place the lamb steaks in a large zip lock bag or bowl. Add the paste and massage the steaks with the paste.
3. Preferably allow the steaks to marinate overnight or give them as long as possible.
4. Preheat a griddle pan and fry each steak for 6-8 minutes, depending on your preference, turning them throughout the cooking process.

Keto Rogan Josh

Lamb Recipe | **Prep Time:** 10 minutes | **Servings:** 4
Per Serving: Kcal: 492, 12g Carbs, 31g Protein, 34g Fat

Ingredients

- 600g Diced Lamb Shoulder
- 30g Ghee (for dairy-free, swap this for Cooking Coconut Oil)
- 100g Shallot
- 400g Chopped Tomatoes
- Large bunch of Fresh Coriander
- 3-4 Garlic Cloves - crushed or finely chopped
- 1 tsp Fresh Ginger - crushed or finely chopped
- 1 tsp Fine Pink / Rock Salt
- 2 tsp Garam Masala
- 2 tsp Ground Coriander
- 1 tsp Turmeric
- 1/4 tsp Cayenne Pepper
- 1/4 tsp Ground Nutmeg
- 1/2 - 1 tsp Chilli Flakes (to taste)

Directions

1. Dice the lamb, place in a bowl, and sprinkle with salt
2. Heat the ghee over medium heat in a large saucepan or wok with a lid.
3. Add the diced lamb and brown for 2 - 3 minutes.
4. Add the shallots and saute over low to medium heat until soft and translucent.
5. Add the garlic and ginger, combine and cook for 1 - 2 minutes.
6. Add all of the spices - Garam Masala, Ground Coriander, Cayenne (avoid if you want a mild dish), Turmeric, and Nutmeg.
7. Fully combine the spices with the meat and add the chopped tomatoes.
8. The combination of spices will create a thick sauce, add a little water, 100 - 200ml water and then cover the dish and cook on low heat for 15 - 20 minutes (depending on the cut of lamb used, this may need to be up to 60 minutes)
9. Remove cover and check the consistency of the sauce. For a thicker sauce, increase the heat and allow to cook for 10 - 15 minutes
10. Add 1/2 - 1 tsp Chilli Flakes and the finishing touch top with chopped Coriander for extra heat.

BEEF RECIPES

Beef and Horseradish Yorkies

Beef Recipe | **Prep Time:** 5 minutes | **Servings:** 12
Per Serving: Kcal: 108, Carbs (net) 3.5 grams, Protein 2.2 grams, Fat 9.5 grams

Ingredients
Batter

- 30g Olive Oil for greasing
- 25g Arrowroot Powder
- 3 Medium Eggs
- 90g Double Cream
- 90g Your favourite milk. I use full-fat Lactose-free
- Seasoning

Other ingredients

- 100g Roast Beef (I used ready sliced from the deli counter)
- 12 tsp Horseradish (1 tsp is approx 7g)
- And any other garnish, I used a shaving of partly cooked carrot and a little rocket (the rocket cannot be frozen)

Directions
The Batter

1. Oven 200C
2. Add a drop of oil to each muffin tin, and pop into the oven till piping hot
3. Add all your batter ingredients to your bullet/mixer and completely blend
4. Divide this mixture between the individual muffins, and pop back in the oven for about 20 to 25 minutes, or until well risen and no soggy bottoms!
5. Allow cooling

Construction

1. Divide your beef slices between the muffins
2. Put 1 tsp / 7g Horseradish in each Yorkie
3. This is purely a choice, but I peeled a carrot for extra color and popped it in the microwave for 2 minutes. Allow cooling. Then peel some slices, roll them up, so it looks like a rose, and place them in the Yorkies
4. The final bit of garnish is something green; I used rocket, but if you're freezing, don't put this on until out of the freezer and ready to eat

Minced Beef & Leek Pie

Beef Recipe | **Prep Time:** 10 minutes | **Servings:** 4
Per Serving: Kcal: 816, 8.5g Carbs, 45g Protein, 66g Fat

Ingredients

Pie Crust

- 1 batch Pie Crust (follow this link to take you to the recipe)

The Filling
- 600g Beef Mince
- 300g Leeks - Small, roughly chopped
- 2 tsp Garlic
- 20g Olive oil
- 10g -15g Arrowroot
- 2 Tbsp Worcestershire sauce
- 20g Tomato puree
- 2 tsp Mixed herbs
- 2 Beef stock cubes
- 150 - 200ml Boiling water (or whatever is needed to give you the right amount of gravy - my husband wanted more, which is why I have upped it to 200ml
- Salt & Pepper (I added 1/2 tsp salt & 1/4 tsp pepper)

Directions
Pie Crust

1. Follow the directions for the Pie Crust recipe (follow this link to take you to the recipe)

Pie Filling

2. Add the oil to a large pan and fry the leeks for about 5-10 minutes, until it's softened but not overly browned
3. Now add the beef mince & garlic and fry until the beef is lightly cooked but not crispy
4. Next, add arrowroot, Worcestershire Sauce, Tomato puree & mixed herbs, and stir through
5. Finally, add the stock cubes & boiling water to the saucepan. Season with salt & pepper. Bring to boil & gently simmer for approx. 15 to 20 minutes.
6. Simmer for longer; if you want to reduce the gravy, or if you like the gravy as it is, but would like it a little thicker, then add a small amount of extra arrowroot to a cup, with a little cold water, mix until smooth and then mix into the pie filling
7. Now pour into your prepared Pie Crust base and go back to the Pie Crust recipe and instruction no.8 onwards
8. Enjoy :-)

Beef Stroganoff

Beef Recipe | **Prep Time:** 10 minutes | **Servings:** 4
Per Serving: Kcal: 329, Carbs (net) 2.7 grams, Protein 35 grams, Fat 20.5 grams

Ingredients
- 30g Butter
- 100g Shallots or Leek, finely chopped
- 250g Mushrooms, sliced
- 15ml Olive Oil
- 600g Diced Beef
- 1 Beef Stock Cube in 100ml Boiling Water
- 1 tsp Dijon Mustard
- 1 tsp Dried Parsley
- 60g Soured Cream / Crème Fraîche

Directions
1. Heat the butter in a large pan or wok with a well-fitting lid over medium heat, and add the onion & mushrooms. Fry for 2-3 minutes until soft.
2. Remove the veg from the pan and add the olive oil.
3. Turn the heat to high and add the beef. Fry for 2-3 minutes, ensuring that all meat has turned brown.
4. Return the onions/mushrooms to the pan and add the beef stock, dijon mustard, and parsley.
5. Heat until the stock begins to boil, reduce the heat to low, and cover the pan with the lid.
6. The dish will generally take between 1- and 2 hours to cook, depending on the meat used. The longer it is allowed to cook over a gentle heat, the more tender the meat will become. Check on the dish every 20-30 minutes to ensure it isn't drying out.
7. Season & add the soured cream when ready to serve.

In a slow cooker:
1. Follow steps 1-3, and then transfer the veg & meat to your slow cooker. Add the beef stock, mustard, and parsley. Allow cooking for 6-8 hours on low or 3-4 hours on high. Season & add the soured cream when ready to serve.

Beef & Tomato Meatloaf

Beef Recipe | **Prep Time:** 10 minutes | **Servings:** 4
Per Serving: Kcal: 284, 3.2g Carbs, 42.9g Protein, 10.8g Fat

Ingredients
- 750g Beef Mince (5% Fat)

- 100g Shallots, diced
- 1 Large Egg
- 75-100g 'Breadcrumbs' - make a 90-second bread or use any other low-carb bread, like our Linseed Bread recipe or Mega Loaf.
- 1 tsp Dried Thyme
- 1 tsp Garlic Powder or 2-3 Garlic Cloves, finely chopped
- 100g Tomato Passata or Homemade Tomato Sauce
- 10ml Worcestershire Sauce
- Salt and Pepper to season

Optional: 100g Pizza Mozzarella (in a block), sliced into thin strips

Directions

2. Preheat the oven to 180°C.
3. Put the beef mince in a large bowl and spend a minute kneading the meat.
4. Create a well in the meat and add all the other ingredients except 25g passata and (if you're using it) the mozzarella.
5. Fully combine all the ingredients - this is best done by hand - and place the mix in a medium loaf tin (ours is 8.5" x 4").
6. Firmly press the mix into the loaf pan. If you're using the mozzarella, split the meat mix in half, press half into the bottom of the pan, and then layer the mozzarella slices in. Press the rest of the meat on top.
7. Bake for 30 minutes.
8. Spoon the remaining passata over the loaf and return to the oven for 10-15 minutes to finish cooking.
9. Allow resting for 10-15 minutes before slicing.

Bolognese Base recipe

Beef Recipe | **Prep Time:** 10 minutes | **Servings:** 4
Per Serving: Kcal: 364, 5.4 g Carbs, 24.4g Protein, 24.4g Fat

Ingredients
- 30g Olive Oil
- 75g Bacon, chopped small
- 100g Leeks, chopped small
- 50g Carrots, chopped small
- 100g Celery, chopped small
- 1tsp Oregano or Mixed Herbs
- 3 Garlic cloves or 1 1/2 tsp garlic powder
- 1 tsp Ketoroma Curry Blend - not enough to taste it, but enough to give an edge :-)
- 500g Beef mince (I like 250g pork & 250g Beef)
- 400g Tinned tomatoes
- 200g Coldwater to rinse out the tinned tomatoes and add to the pan

- 1tsp Salt
- Freshly ground pepper
- 15g 85% Dark Chocolate (this is included in the macros, but it is optional - it makes the meat sauce a lot richer)
- 15g Basil, to decorate

Directions
1. Add the olive oil to a large non-stick saucepan and gently heat.
2. Add the chopped bacon, leeks, carrots & celery and cook for about 5 minutes until softened.
3. Add the garlic, herbs, curry blend, and meat to the saucepan. Carry on frying until the meat has browned for around 5 - 10 minutes.
4. Add the tinned tomatoes, water (I use the water to clean out the tomato tins), salt & pepper.
5. Now simmer for about 30 - 45 minutes, or until you're happy that the sauce has reduced to a beautiful, silky sauce
6. Stir in the dark chocolate chunks until melted.
7. And finally, top with basil leaves, or sprinkle on when serving.

Bone Broth

Beef Recipe | **Prep Time:** 10 minutes | **Servings:** 4
Per Serving: Kcal: 108, Carbs (net) 3.5 grams, Protein 2.2 grams, Fat 9.5 grams

Ingredients
- 750g Meaty Bones (we get these from Morrisons)
- 2 Marrow Bones
- 2 Medium Carrots
- 1 small bunch of Flat Leaf Parsley or any other fresh herb of choice
- 1.5-2 liters of Boiling Water
- 1 tsp Pink Himalayan / Rock / Sea Salt

Directions
1. Pan-fry the bones and carrots in a large frying pan over medium/high heat. We used the Sear function on the Ninja Foodi.
2. Once the bones have browned on each side, transfer all ingredients to a slow cooker and cover the bones with boiling water.
3. Add the salt and parsley and allow to cook for a minimum of 24 hours.

4. Remove the meat and carrots but leave the bones to cook for 12 hours. Refrigerate the meat in a container to allow any fat to solidify. Once cooled, you'll be able to remove the fat from the meat quickly.
5. Remove the layer of fat from the stock, place any fat from the meat into a pan, and heat over medium heat. Allow any water to cook away - it'll stop spitting once all the liquid has been cooked away.
6. Allow the fat to cool and strain through a stainless steel sieve to remove any food and store it in the fridge. This fat can be used when roasting vegetables or frying.
7. Reheat the stock and reduce over a gentle heat for 15-20 minutes.
8. The stock can be stored in the fridge. When you want a cup of bone broth, take about 100ml out and reheat.

Cauliflower Bomb

Beef Recipe | **Prep Time:** 14 minutes | **Servings:** 4
Per Serving: Kcal: 378, 11.5g Carbs, 37. g Protein, 18.9g Fat

Ingredients
- 600g (1 medium) Cauliflower
- 500g Beef Mince (we used 5% fat) - this can be swapped for any other mince
- 50g Shallots, finely chopped
- 20g Tomato Puree
- 2 tsp Smoked Paprika
- 1 tsp Garlic Powder
- 60g Mature Cheddar
- For an extra kick, add a red chilli to the meat!

The Sauce
- 400g Tinned Chopped Tomatoes
- 1/2 tsp Salt
- 1 tsp Dried Oregano
- Optional: 60g Mascarpone

Directions
1. Preheat the oven to 180°C.
2. Remove as many of the outer leaves from the cauliflower as you want - the leaves can be eaten, so they don't have to be removed.
3. To ensure the cauliflower isn't too crunchy after being baked, it's best to steam it for 10-15 minutes first, or place it in a large microwaveable bowl with a well-fitting lid and add 50ml water to the bowl. Microwave on 70-80% power for 5 minutes. You want the cauliflower to be hot but not cooked.

4. While the cauliflower is steaming, mix the meat, shallots, tomato puree, and spices in a large bowl, and this can also be pulsed in a food processor.
5. If making the sauce, add the tin of tomatoes, seasonings, and cauliflower to a deep casserole dish. Take the meat mix and cover the cauliflower. Press firmly all around and either cover with a lid or foil to create a seal.
6. Bake for 25-30 minutes.
7. Remove the lid/foil and sprinkle the cheese over the top. Bake for a further 10 minutes or until the cheese has melted.
8. Lift the cauliflower and put it on a serving plate. Stir the sauce to combine all the flavours from the meat (at this stage, you could use a hand blender to create a smooth sauce and even add the mascarpone to make it creamy). Enjoy!

Chilli Con Carne in Ninja Foodi

Beef Recipe | **Prep Time:** 14 minutes | **Servings:** 4
Per Serving: Kcal: 366, Carbs (net) 7 grams, Protein 27.2 grams, Fat 25.7 grams

Ingredients
- 2 tbsp (30ml) Olive Oil
- 450-500g Beef Mince (15%)
- 100g Shallots, chopped
- 1 tsp Chilli Powder
- 1 tsp Ground Cumin
- 3 tbsp (45g) Tomato Puree
- 400g Tinned Chopped Tomatoes
- 1 Beef Stock Cube with 300ml Boiling Water
- Fresh coriander - chopped

Optional: Soured Cream & Fresh coriander for serving

Directions
1. Using the sauté function on the Ninja, heat the olive oil in the central pan.
2. Add the chopped shallots to the pan.
3. Once softened, add the mincemeat and cook for 5 mins, until browned.
4. Add the spices and tomato puree and cook for another minute.
5. Add the chopped tomatoes and stock, and bring to a boil.
6. Reduce the heat and simmer for around 40 minutes until the sauce is reduced and thick.
7. 5 minutes before the end, add the coriander and season to taste.
8. Serve with swede rice/cauliflower rice with soured cream and coriander.

Chunky Beef Chilli

Beef Recipe | **Prep Time:** 10 minutes | **Servings:** 4
Per Serving: Kcal: 372, Carbs (net) 7.4 grams, Protein 35.7 grams, Fat 22.3 grams

Ingredients
- 40ml Olive Oil
- 80g Shallots
- 600g Diced Beef
- 200g Aubergine
- 80g Red Pepper
- 1 Beef Stock Cube in 200ml boiling water (if you're using a slow cooker, leave the stock cube as it is - sees instructions at the end of the method)
- 400g (1 tin) Chopped Tomatoes
- 1 Medium Hot Chilli or 1/2 tsp Chilli Flakes
- 2 tsp Garam Masala
- 1/2 tsp Ground Cumin

Optional: 100g Soured Cream

Directions
1. Heat the oil in a large pan or wok over medium heat. Dice or slice the shallots and add them to the pan. Fry for 2-3 minutes until soft (not brown).
2. Turn the heat to high and add the diced beef. Cook on high until the beef has been browned on all sides.
3. Slice or dice the aubergine and pepper and add these to the pan. Cook for 1-2 minutes on high heat.
4. Add the beef stock and bring it back to boil.
5. Stir in the chopped tomatoes and spiced, return to boil, then reduce the heat to allow the dish to simmer for 45-60 minutes.
6. Season and stir in the soured cream when ready to serve.

In a slow cooker:
1. Follow steps 1-3, and then transfer to your slow cooker. Crumble a stock cube over the dish without the water and add the tomatoes and spices. Allow cooking for 6-8 hours on low. Season and add the soured cream when ready to serve.

Cottage Pie

Beef Recipe | **Prep Time:** 20 minutes | **Servings:** 4
Per Serving: Kcal: 351, Carbs (net) 9.8 grams, Protein 36 grams, Fat 19 grams

Ingredients
- 40g Butter
- 100g Leeks
- 200g Courgette
- 500g Minced Beef (5%)
- 1 Beef Stock Cube in 200ml Boiling Water
- 800g (1 medium head) Cauliflower Florets
- 1/2 tsp thyme
- 40g Soft Cream Cheese
- Seasoning to taste

Directions
2. Preheat the oven to 180°C.
3. Heat the butter in a large pan or wok over medium heat. Dice or slice the leek and add to the pan. Fry for 2-3 minutes until soft, not brown.
4. Add the diced courgettes and fry for 2-3 minutes.
5. Either remove the leek/courgettes from the pan or push them to the side. Add the minced beef.
6. Cook the beef until brown and combine with the leek/courgette.
7. Add the beef stock. Bring to boil, then reduce the heat to simmer uncovered.
8. Break the cauliflower into small florets. Boil for 8-10minutes in a separate pan and drain well. Return them to the pan and add the seasoning and cream cheese. Mash them together.
9. Once the meat stock has reduced, transfer the mix to an ovenproof dish and top with the cauliflower mash.
10. Finish in the oven for 20-25 minutes to allow the mash to brown.
11. Serve with some fried kale... proper winter grub!

Crispy Chilli Beef

Beef Recipe | **Prep Time:** 10 minutes | **Servings:** 2
Per Serving: Kcal: 416, Carbs (net) 5.7 grams, Protein 64.7 grams, Fat 14.5 grams

Ingredients
- 340g Beef Medallions
- 50g Spring Onions
- 20g Ginger Root
- 3 Garlic Cloves
- 1 or 2 Birds Eye Chilli
- 10ml Sesame Oil
- 10ml White Rice Vinegar
- 20ml Liquid Aminos (this is a soy sauce replacement)
- 20g Homemade Tomato Sauce (we use Sandie's Ketchup)
- 1 Egg

- 40g Egg White Powder (we get this from MyProtein)
- 200-300g Cooking Coconut Oil (this has no taste - we use the KTC brand from Morrisons) or Lard
- 10g Coriander

Directions

1. Tenderise the beef with a meat tenderizing mallet or a rolling pin.
2. Slice the beef into very thin strips and place in a bowl suitable to marinate the meat for several hours overnight.
3. In a bowl, mix the egg, 5ml of sesame oil, and 10ml liquid amino. Pour the mix over the beef and allow to marinade.

Only prepare the next stage when you are ready to cook the beef.

1. Finely chop the Garlic, Ginger, Chilli, Coriander Stalks (save the leaves for dressing the dish at the end), and Spring Onions and set them aside for cooking.
2. In a large wok / deep pan, add the cooking coconut oil/lard and bring to 200°C.
3. Add around half of the egg white powder to a large mixing bowl. Lift about half of the beef from the marinade, shake off any excess and add to the protein powder. Shake the bowl to coat the meat in the powder fully. This may clump together initially but continue shaking, and the beef will start to separate. If you feel it needs a bit of egg white powder, add another 10g and shake again.
4. Ensure you have a slotted spoon and a dish ready with some kitchen towel before cooking the beef.
5. The cooking process takes seconds, and you don't want to overload your work. Take only half of the beef from the powder and carefully add it to the hot oil.
6. This should immediately burst into life and almost instantly go golden brown. Using a metal slotted spoon, carefully move the beef around in the hot oil to ensure all sides are cooked, and this will take less than 20 seconds.
7. Remove this batch, place it in a bowl with a kitchen towel, and repeat it until all beef is coated and cooked.
8. You can either remove the hot oil from the pan (ensure the container you will use is suitable for hot oil (Pyrex or ceramic dish only) or start the next process with a new pan.
9. Add 5ml sesame oil to the pan and heat over medium heat. Add the garlic, ginger, chilli, and spring onion mix and gently fry in the oil.

There are 2 options at this point - Option 1:

1. Once the garlic mix has started to go golden brown, turn the heat to complete and add the coated beef into the pan. Quick fry the beef is combining the garlic mix throughout.

Option 2 - for a slightly sticky chilli beef:

2. In a small bowl, mix the tomato sauce, 10ml liquid aminos, and 10ml rice wine vinegar and add to the garlic chill mix in the pan.
3. Turn the heat to full, quickly stir the sauce in and then add the beef to the pan combining as much of the beef in the sauce.

Keto Goulash

Beef Recipe | **Prep Time:** 15 minutes | **Servings:** 4
Per Serving: Kcal: 400, Carbs (net) 8 grams, Protein 41 grams, Fat 24 grams

Ingredients
- 40ml Olive Oil
- 700g Lean Diced Beef
- 100g Shallots, diced
- 3-4 Garlic Cloves, chopped
- 80g (1 medium) Red Pepper, diced
- 80g Fresh Tomatoes, diced
- 20g Flat Leaf Parsley, chopped
- 2 tsp Smoked Paprika
- 300ml/g Beef Stock (homemade bone broth or Bovril cube)
- 100g Soured Cream (alternatively use mascarpone or, for a dairy-free version, coconut milk)

Directions
1. Heat the oil over medium heat in a large pan with a well-fitting lid as this dish will need to cook for around 2 hours. Alternatively, you can transfer to a slow cooker once the beef stock has been added. If using a Ninja Foodi, use the sear function until the beef stock has been added, and then switch to slow cook.

2. Add the diced beef, shallots, and garlic to the hot oil and fry until the meat has started to brown. Cover with a lid and allow to cook for 2-3 minutes.
3. Add the peppers, tomatoes, parsley, and paprika, combine with the meat and cook for 2-3 minutes.
4. Add the beef stock and increase the heat to bring it to a boil.
5. Cover over low heat for at least 90 minutes to make the meat tender, or transfer everything into a slow cooker (high for around 4 hours or low for around 8 hours).
6. When you are ready to serve the dish, add the soured cream.

Keto Lasagne

Beef Recipe | **Prep Time:** 20 minutes | **Servings:** 4
Per Serving: Kcal: 515, Carbs (net) 7.7 grams, Protein 32.1 grams, Fat 39.3 grams

Ingredients
- 30ml Olive Oil
- 80g Shallots
- 500g Beef Steak Mince (around 10% fat)
- 1 tsp Garlic Puree or 1/2 tsp Garlic Powder
- 1 tsp Mixed Italian Herbs
- 400g (1 tin) Chopped Tomatoes
- 100g Soured Cream
- 60g Mascarpone Cheese
- 400g Aubergine
- 60g Mature Cheddar Cheese

Directions
1. Preheat the oven to 200°C.
2. Dice the shallots and lightly fry them in the oil over medium heat for 3-5 minutes to soften but not brown.
3. Break the minced beef up over the onions and cook thoroughly over medium-high heat until all of the mince is brown.
4. Add the garlic, herbs, and the tin of chopped tomatoes.
5. Cook for 5 minutes over medium heat until the tomatoes begin to bubble. Add seasoning to taste and remove the pan from the heat.
6. Add the soured cream and mascarpone cheese over gentle heat in a small saucepan. Mix them until smooth.
7. Pour half the meat mixture into an ovenproof dish and layer with sliced aubergine, more meat, and the other aubergines.
8. Top with the cheese sauce and sprinkle grated cheddar on top.

9. Bake for around 30 minutes or until golden.

Meatball & Garlic Bread Bake

Beef Recipe | **Prep Time:** 10 minutes | **Servings:** 4
Per Serving: Kcal: 548, 6.6g Carbs, 38.9g Protein, 29.9g Fat

Ingredients
- 500g Beef Mince (we use 15%)
- 100g Shallots, finely chopped
- 1 Large Egg
- 30g Butter
- 400g Tinned Chopped Tomatoes or Passata
- Seasoning/spices of choice, e.g., one chilli, finely chopped, garlic powder, mixed herbs, etc
- 2 Garlic Cloves, finely chopped/crushed
- Around 160g 'Bread.' We used Linseed Bread - you could also make two 90 second pieces of bread.
- 40g Grated Parmesan (adjust to taste)

Directions
1. Preheat the oven to 180°C.
2. Start by thinly slicing the bread and melting 15g of butter in a small dish.
3. Mix the butter with the sliced/crushed garlic, and then brush this butter over the slices of bread. Allow the bread to soak up the butter.
4. To make the meatballs: add the beef mince, 40 chopped shallots, an egg, and any spices/seasoning to a bowl. Mix thoroughly.
5. Form 12 meatballs from the mixture, rolling the mix in your hand. Heat a pan over medium heat and add the meatballs, frying to color all sides. We find we don't need any added oil due to the fat content of the meat, but add some butter/cooking coconut oil if needed.
6. Once the meatballs are brown (they don't need to be fully cooked as they're being baked), transfer them to an oven dish and return the pan to the heat.
7. Add the remaining 15g butter and 50g shallots. Fry over a gentle heat to soften the shallots.
8. Add the tomatoes (blitz chopped tomatoes first if you prefer a smooth sauce), bring to the boil, then simmer for 5-10 minutes to reduce slightly.
9. Pour the tomato sauce over the meatballs in the oven-proof dish.
10. Tear up the garlic bread and place the pieces on top of the meatballs & sauce.

11. Finally, sprinkle the grated parmesan on top, then place the dish in the oven to bake for around 15 minutes, until the bread is nice & toasty and the cheese is golden.

Spiced Up Beef Burgers

Beef Recipe | **Prep Time:** 10 minutes | **Servings:** 4
Per Serving: Kcal: 262, Carbs (net) 2.5 grams, Protein 26 grams, Fat 16 gram

Ingredients
- 20g Butter or Olive Oil
- 100g Shallots, finely chopped if not using a food processor
- 100g Red Pepper, finely chopped if not using a food processor
- 500g Aberdeen Angus Beef Mince (steak mince, 5-10% fat)
- 1 tsp Hot Chilli Powder
- 2 tsp Garam Masala
- Salt & Pepper to taste

Directions
1. Heat the butter/oil in a medium pan and fry the shallots & pepper over gentle heat for 6-8 minutes to slowly brown. Remove from the heat and allow to cool a little.
2. The burger mix can be made in a food processor or mixed by hand. Add all ingredients to a bowl/food processor and mix well.
3. Divide the mix into 4 or 8, depending on how thick you want each burger.
4. Use a burger press or mold the mix in your hands, pressing firmly.
5. Heat a skillet pan or good non-stick frying pan over medium heat. Depending on the thickness of the burgers, fry for around 3-5 minutes on each side to ensure they are fully cooked.

Tex Mex Beef Chilli

Beef Recipe | **Prep Time:** 10 minutes | **Servings:** 4
Per Serving: Kcal: 431, Carbs (net) 6.7 grams, Protein 33.4 grams, Fat 30.3 grams

Ingredients
- 30g Butter or Olive Oil
- 100g Leeks, finely chopped
- 100g Green Pepper, diced
- 100g Aubergine or Courgette, finely diced
- 500g Minced Beef (10-12% fat)
- 1/2 - 1 tsp Chilli Flakes
- 1/2 - 1 tsp Paprika

- 1-2 tsp Garam Masala
- 200g (half tin) Chopped Tomatoes
- 50g Soured Cream
- 100g Grated Mozzarella

If making stuffed peppers:
- 8 Bell Peppers (green are lowest in carbs, but red also works well)

Directions
1. If you're making stuffed peppers, preheat the oven to 180°C
2. Melt the butter/oil in a saucepan and fry the leek, pepper, and aubergine/courgette for 3-5 minutes over medium heat until the veg softens but does not brown.
3. Remove the veg from the pan and set it aside.
4. Return the pan to the heat and break up the mince as you add it. Cook over medium-high heat for around 5 minutes or until all the meat has browned.
5. Add the veg back to the pan, combine, then add all spices, tomatoes, and soured cream.
6. Allow the dish to heat through thoroughly and either reduce the heat & cover with a lid for 15-20 minutes if you are going to serve this with cauliflower/broccoli rice (add the mozzarella when serving), or place the chilli in bell peppers in an ovenproof dish and bake for 35-45 minutes. Remove the stuffed peppers from the oven and add the cheese before returning them to the oven for 10 minutes.

Keto Winter Stew

Beef Recipe | **Prep Time:** 10 minutes | **Servings:** 4
Per Serving: Kcal: 426, Carbs (net) 12 grams, Fat 16 grams, Protein 37 grams

Ingredients
- 1kg Gammon Joint (Smoked or Unsmoked) - trim the fat off and cube the joint into bite-size pieces. Alternatively, use Diced Pork Shoulder or Diced Stewing Beef
- 400g Diced Swede or Celeriac
- 200g Diced Celery
- 200g Diced Carrots
- 200g Diced Courgettes or Aubergines
- 200g Diced Leeks or Shallots
- 50g Unsalted Butter
- 250ml Vegetable Stock - Homemade is best
- 400g Chopped Tomatoes

- 1 tsp Smoked Paprika
- 1 tsp Ground Cumin
- 1 tsp Ground Coriander
- 1 tsp Arrowroot Powder - Optional
- 60g Mascarpone Cheese / Soured Cream Optional

Directions

1. Melt the butter in a large stockpot over medium heat and add the Gammon (meat) cubes. Cook for 2 - 3 minutes to brown, add the diced swede, and combine with the meat.
2. Transfer the meat and swede into a slow cooker leaving the meat juices/butter in the pan.
3. Add the stock, tomatoes, and spices to the meat & swede in the slow cooker, and cover. Set to either high for 4 hrs or low for around 8 hrs.
4. The rest of the vegetables can be prepared straight away and allowed to cool to add to the stew later or cooked later closer to serving time.
5. Using the butter/meat juices - add all of the remaining vegetables and sweat down over low/medium heat for 10 minutes.
6. Add these vegetables to the stew near the end of the cooking time and combine.
7. Stir through the mascarpone / soured cream, or If you want to thicken the sauce, mix the arrowroot with a tablespoon of cold water and mix with a paste.
8. Add the arrowroot paste to the stew and stir through.
9. Season to taste and serve.

CHEESE RECIPES

Cauliflower & Broccoli Cheese

Cheese Recipe | **Prep Time:** 10 minutes | **Servings:** 4
Per Serving: Kcal: 448, Carbs 7.9 grams, Protein 13 grams, Fat 40.1 grams

Ingredients

- 20g Butter
- 80g Fresh Leeks, finely chopped
- 2-3 Garlic Cloves, finely chopped
- 400g Cauliflower Florets
- 200g Broccoli Florets
- 100g Mascarpone Cheese (or cream cheese)
- 125g Double Cream (or sour cream)
- 100g Mature Cheddar (or other grated cheese)
- Optional: 300g Bacon Lardons

Directions

1. Preheat the oven to 180°C.
2. Melt the butter in a large saucepan over medium heat and add the chopped leeks and garlic.
3. Add this now and cook for 2-3 minutes if including the bacon.
4. Break the cauliflower and broccoli into bite-sized pieces, rinse, and add to the saucepan. Cover the pan and allow to cook on medium heat for 5 minutes.
5. Add the mascarpone and cream (or alternatives) and gently combine.
6. Transfer the contents of the dish into an oven-proof dish. Sprinkle evenly with grated cheddar and bake for 30-40 minutes or until golden brown.

Celeriac Dauphinoise with Garlic

Cheese Recipe | **Prep Time:** 10 minutes | **Servings:** 4
Per Serving: Kcal: 304, Carbs (net) 5.6 grams, Protein 9.2 grams, Fat 26.3 grams

Ingredients

- 500g Celeriac, thinly sliced
- 100g/ml Double Cream
- 300g Crème Fraîche
- 1/4 tsp Ground Turmeric
- 1 Large Garlic Clove, chopped as finely as possible
- 100g Mature Cheddar Cheese, grated
- 100g Pre-Grated Mozzarella
- 25g Parmesan Cheese, grated
- Freshly Ground Black Pepper
- Salt to taste

Directions

1. Preheat the oven to 170°C.
2. Parboil the celeriac in salted water for 15 minutes. Drain and allow to cool slightly.
3. Add the cream, crème fraîche, and turmeric to a bowl and mix.
4. Begin to layer the celeriac in a baking dish, sprinkling some of the garlic on top. Then add some of the cream mixture, a touch of salt & pepper, and some of the grated cheddar & mozzarella.
5. Repeat step 4 until you run out of celeriac. Ensure you have some of the cream mixture and grated cheese for the next step.
6. Finish off the dish with the remaining cream mixture and grated cheese. Then add the grated parmesan on top to give it a nice crunch.
7. Bake for 40 minutes or remove when golden.

Keto Chaffle

Cheese Recipe | **Prep Time:** 2 minutes | **Servings:** 2
Per Serving: Kcal: 218, Carbs (net) 1.5 grams, Protein 18.4 grams, Fat 15 grams

Ingredients
- 75g Grated Mozzarella (pre-grated)
- 3 Large Eggs
- Spices & Seasoning to taste - e.g., Garlic Powder & Italian Herbs

Directions
1. Beat the eggs and add the grated mozzarella and spices/seasoning. Mix until thoroughly combined.
2. Pour half of the mix into the waffle press (use a quarter of the mix if you have a smaller waffle maker). Cook for 1-2 minutes until golden brown.

Cheese & Leek Splat Filling

Cheese Recipe | **Prep Time:** 15 minutes | **Servings:** 4
Per Serving: Kcal: 324, Carbs (net) 3.5 grams, Protein 17.4 grams, Fat 26.1 grams

Ingredients
- 160g Leeks, chopped finely
- 160g Cheddar Cheese, grated
- 40g Soft Cream Cheese
- 15ml/g Butter / Olive Oil
- 1 batch of MKD - see recipe

Directions
1. Add oil or butter to the pan and heat up

2. Add the leeks to the pan and fry gently until thoroughly cooked.
3. Take the heated pan and add the grated cheddar and soft cream cheese.
4. Mix well, allow to cool slightly, and then place in the freezer while you make the MKD.
5. Head to the MKD recipe to make the pastry and complete your 'splat' :)

Cheese-Loaf & Burgers

Cheese Recipe | **Prep Time:** 10 minutes | **Servings:** 2
Per Serving: Kcal: 484, Carbs (net) 5.9 grams, Protein 30.2 grams, Fat 36.5 grams

Ingredients
- 200g Halloumi / Grilling Cheese
- 50g Red Pepper, diced
- 50g Courgette, diced
- 25g Shallots / Leek, finely chopped
- 2 Large Eggs
- 10g Coconut Flour (alternatively, use 10g Psyllium Husk - see the description above for more details)
- 15g Chopped Fresh Herbs, e.g., Coriander, Thyme, Parsley
- 1/2 tsp Garlic Powder / Chilli Flakes / Smoked Paprika - you choose!

Directions
1. Preheat the oven to 180°C.
2. Blitz the halloumi/grilling cheese in a food processor to a fine crumb.
3. In a large bowl, combine all of the ingredients - you could do this in the food processor if you wanted finely diced veg, but don't over-process it as it will go watery.
4. Place the mix in a lined small loaf tin (ours is 9cm x 15cm) and bake for 30 minutes or until golden and firm. Or, divide the mix into little round dishes (2.5") and bake for 15 minutes.

Cheesy Seed Crackers

Cheese Recipe | **Prep Time:** 12 minutes | **Servings:** 8
Per Serving: Kcal: 126, 1g Carbs, 6g Protein, 10g Fat

Ingredients
- 140g Mixed Seeds (we buy bags of mixed seeds - pumpkin, sunflower, linseed/flax & sesame)
- 5g Psyllium Husk (the whole husks)
- 1 Large Egg
- 30g Grated Cheddar (or another strong cheese like Manchego or Gouda)

- Seasoning to taste

Directions
1. Preheat the oven to 180°C.
2. Add all of the ingredients to a bowl and combine. Allow the mix to rest for 5-10 minutes - it will begin to thicken as the psyllium husk absorbs moisture.
3. Line an oven tray with greaseproof baking paper and spread the mix out as thin as possible. Score the crackers before baking - this will help separate them once baked.
4. Bake for 15 minutes, then flip the crackers over. Bake for another 10 minutes to make them crispy on both sides.
5. Break the crackers apart along the score lines, allow them to fully cool, and store them in an airtight container in the cupboard or fridge.

Cheesy Soda Bread

Cheese Recipe | **Prep Time:** 15 minutes | **Servings:** 8
Per Serving: Kcal: 233, Carbs (net) 3.9 grams, Protein 9.8 grams, Fat 19.5 grams

Ingredients
- 100g Cheddar Cheese, grated
- 30g Melted Butter (if you're making the leek soda bread, you'll need 10g for frying the leeks, and the other 20g will be added to the mix)
- 3 Large Eggs
- 15ml Apple Cider Vinegar
- 45g Chia Seeds
- 125g Ground Almonds or Milled Seeds (e.g., milled linseed)
- 1/2 tsp Bicarbonate of Soda
- 1/4 tsp Sea Salt / Pink Himalayan Salt
- Optional: 150g Leeks, chopped

Directions
1. Preheat the oven to 180°C.
2. If you're adding leeks, start by melting 10g in a small pan and frying the leeks for 5 minutes to soften.
3. Melt the remaining butter (or all of the butter if not adding leeks) in a large mixing bowl and allow to cool.
4. Add the eggs, chia seeds, and apple cider vinegar to the butter and whisk.
5. Allow resting for 5-10 minutes.
6. Add the rest of the ingredients (including the fried leeks if you're using them) and mix well. The mix should be gloopy but not to the point that you can't mold it. Having wet hands will help you handle the dough.

7. Place the mix on a lined baking tray and roughly mold it into a circular shape. You can also make these as individual rolls.
8. Bake for 30-35 minutes (less if making rolls - around 15-20 minutes). Ensure the bread is firm before removing it from the oven.

Crispy Pancakes

Cheese Recipe | **Prep Time:** 15 minutes | **Servings:** 6
Per Serving: Kcal: 180, Carbs (net) 4.1 grams, Protein 10.6 grams, Fat 13.3 grams

Ingredients
- Bean Sauce
- 400g Tinned Tomatoes
- 4 tsp Malt Vinegar
- 2 tsp Truvia / Natvia / Pure Via Sweetener
- 1 tsp Kashmiri Chilli
- 1/2 tsp Mixed Spice
- Salt & Pepper
- Beans - 1 batch

Directions
1. Preheat the oven to 180°C
2. If you have a Nutri-bullet or equivalent, put all the sauce ingredients in and blend
3. If not, put it straight into the saucepan, and use a hand blender. Blend until super smooth
4. In a saucepan, bring the smooth bean sauce to boil and then turn down and simmer on low heat for about 10 minutes
5. Meanwhile, while the sauce is simmering, make the MKD as per the instructions.
6. If you like playing with playdough, you'll love this bit! 2 choices here. Either break off small pieces and roll into balls or roll into a thin sausage and cut into small bean-sized chunks, and I do a bit of both.
7. Place your 'Beans' on a lined baking tray and bake for 12 minutes
8. Add the beans to the sauce if you're eating straight away; otherwise, store them separately from the sauce in the fridge.

Halloumi Balti Curry

Cheese Recipe | **Prep Time:** 15 minutes | **Servings:** 4
Per Serving: Kcal: 447, Carbs (net) 9.2 grams, Protein 27.9 grams, Fat 33.1 grams

Ingredients

- 20ml Olive Oil
- 100g Shallots, diced
- 100g (1 medium) Green Bell Pepper, chopped
- 10g Garlic Puree / 2-3 Garlic Cloves
- 10g Ginger Puree / 1-inch cube Fresh Ginger
- 1 tsp Mustard Seeds
- 1/2 tsp Ground Fenugreek or 1 tsp Dried Fenugreek
- 1/2 - 1 tsp Kashmiri Chilli
- 1/2 tsp Ground Turmeric
- 400g Tinned Chopped Tomatoes
- 450g Halloumi / Grilling Cheese, chopped into bite-sized pieces
- A handful of fresh coriander, chopped

Directions
1. Heat the olive oil over medium heat in a large frying pan/wok, and add the diced onion & pepper. Fry for 5 minutes over medium heat to soften but not brown.
2. Add the garlic, ginger, and mustard seeds and fry for around 3-4 minutes - the seeds will start to pop open after a couple of minutes.
3. Add the dried spices and fry for another 1-2 minutes.
4. Add the tinned tomatoes & water.
5. Bring the sauce to a boil and add the halloumi.
6. Allow simmering with a lid/cover for 15-20 minutes over medium heat.
7. Remove the cover and turn up the heat for the final few minutes to allow the sauce to thicken.
8. Sprinkle with some freshly chopped coriander and serve with cauliflower rice or salad.

Halloumi Bolognese

Cheese Recipe | **Prep Time:** 10 minutes | **Servings:** 4
Per Serving: Kcal: 497, Carbs (net) 10.1 grams, Protein 27.9 grams, Fat 37.8 grams

Ingredients
- 40ml Olive Oil
- 450g Halloumi / Grilling Cheese, diced
- 100g Shallots, diced
- 100g Red Pepper, diced
- 250g Courgette, diced
- 150g Aubergine, diced
- 400g Chopped Tomatoes
- 1 tsp Garlic Powder
- 3-4 Fresh Basil Leaves

Directions

1. Heat the olive oil over medium heat in a large frying pan/wok. Add all the vegetables and halloumi and fry for 2-3 minutes. Keep everything moving as the halloumi will stick to the pan quite easily.
2. Once the vegetables soften and brown, add the chopped tomatoes, basil, and garlic powder.
3. Stir, bring to boil, and then reduce the heat. Allow simmering with a lid/cover for 15-20 minutes over medium heat.
4. Remove the cover and turn up the heat for the final few minutes to allow some of the moisture to cook away.

Halloumi Fries

Cheese Recipe | **Prep Time:** 10 minutes | **Servings:** 4
Per Serving: Kcal: 157, Carbs (net) 0.4 grams, Protein 11 grams, Fat 12.3 grams

Ingredients
- 200g Halloumi / Grilling Cheese
- If frying: 250g Lard / Cooking Coconut Oil (lots of this will be leftover)

Directions
1. Cut the halloumi into chips. Don't make them too thin.
2. Dry the halloumi on some kitchen towels.

If frying:
1. Heat the oil gradually over medium heat in a saucepan. The oil needs to be hot but not smoking before you use it. To test if the oil is hot enough, dip the end of one of the fries in the oil, and it should sizzle around the cheese.
2. Carefully place a couple of the fries in the oil. Don't add them all simultaneously, as this can cause the oil to bubble over. After a few seconds, add the next couple. The fries will only take 20-30 seconds to turn golden brown. As you add more fries to the oil, you may need to increase the heat slightly.
3. Remove the fries and place them on a kitchen towel to remove any excess oil.

Air fryer:
1. Preheat the air fryer to 200°C and cook the fries until golden - times will vary depending on the machine.

Crunchy Mozzarella Sticks

Cheese Recipe | **Prep Time:** 5 minutes | **Servings:** 8

Per Serving: Kcal: 144, Carbs (net) 1.1 grams, Protein 10.6 grams, Fat 10.5 grams

Ingredients

- 250g Hard Block Mozzarella - labeled Pizza Mozzarella
- 25g Coconut Flour
- 2 Eggs, mixed up with a fork
- 50 - 60g Pork Scratchings
- Seasoning

Directions

2. Preheat the oven to 200°C.
3. Slice up your mozzarella into sticks/chips
4. Blitz the pork scratchings to resemble bread crumbs, and pop them into a bowl
5. Line up 3 bowls, 1 with coconut flour (seasoned), 1 with mixed up egg, and finally, your blitzed pork scratchings
6. Prepare to get sticky fingers for the next 5 minutes!
7. Coat the mozzarella sticks in the coconut flour, then egg, then the pork scratching, and lay on a lined baking tray, with a small gap between each one
8. Bake until golden brown and crispy (approx 10 - 15 minutes)
9. If freezing, freeze uncooked and cook fresh

Olive & Feta Salad

Cheese Recipe | **Prep Time:** 5 minutes | **Servings:** 2
Per Serving: Kcal: 287, Carbs (net) 0.9 grams, Protein 10.7 grams, Fat 26.4 grams

Ingredients

- 1 Bag of Rocket Leaves (80-100g)
- 100g Feta cheese, chopped into bite-size cubes
- 50g Olives of your choice
- 1-2 Garlic Cloves
- A pinch of Pink Himalayan / Rock / Sea Salt
- 25ml Extra Virgin Olive Oil
- Juice half a lemon
- Ground Pepper

Directions

1. Add all the rocket, olives, and feta and mix in a bowl.
2. In a pestle and mortar, crush the garlic with salt.
3. Add the olive oil and lemon juice to the garlic.
4. Mix and now add the salt and pepper to taste. Lots of black pepper isn't essential, but it can make the salad slightly spicy.

5. Pour the lemon mixture over the salad, mix through, and eat straight away. The salad can be prepared in advance - just don't add the dressing until you are ready to eat.

Saag Paneer

Cheese Recipe | **Prep Time:** 10 minutes | **Servings:** 4
Per Serving: Kcal: 255, Carbs (net) 3.9 grams, Protein 9.5 grams, Fat 22.3 grams

Ingredients

- 100g Shallots, sliced
- 1 inch Ginger, crushed
- 4-5 Garlic Cloves, crushed
- 25g Butter
- 2 Medium (around 40g) Tomatoes, diced
- 150g Paneer Cheese, cubed
- 15ml/g Olive Oil or Cooking Coconut Oil (this has no flavour or taste - we use this one)
- 1/4 tsp Ground Turmeric
- 1/2 tsp Hot Chilli Powder
- 15g Pine Nuts
- 1 Bag (around 250g) of Spinach
- 1 tsp Dried Fenugreek Leaves
- 15g Greek or Greek Style Yogurt
- Chopped fresh coriander for garnish

Directions

1. In a medium-sized pan with a lid, begin to soften the shallots in butter but don't let them color. Use the lid to keep in the steam.
2. After 5 minutes, add the ginger & garlic. Keep the lid on, allowing the steam to heat the spices.
3. Add the tomatoes and cook for around 5 minutes.
4. Add the turmeric, chilli powder, and pine nuts and cook for 2 minutes.
5. Wash the spinach in a colander - don't worry about drying it.
6. Heat the coconut oil or olive oil in a frying pan and fry the paneer cubes until golden brown. Set aside.
7. Add the spinach and dried fenugreek to the spices and wilt down. Add the paneer, and stir until the spinach is cooked.
8. Season with salt and more chilli if required.
9. Empty into a serving dish, garnish with a Greek / Greek-style yogurt dollop, chopped coriander, and a light sprinkling of chilli powder.

BREAD RECIPES

2 Minute Bread

Bread Recipe | **Prep Time:** 1 minute | **Servings:** 1
Per Serving: Kcal: 110, Carbs (net) 2.6 grams, Protein 8.1 grams, Fat 5.8 grams

Ingredients
- 1 Large Egg
- 1 tsp Coconut Flour
- 1 tsp Psyllium Husk
- 2 tsp Apple Cider Vinegar
- 1/4 tsp Xanthan Gum
- 1/2 tsp Baking Powder
- Seasoning to taste

Directions
1. Mix all of the ingredients in a microwaveable dish. This can be a ramekin, wide mug, or microwavable tub.
2. Microwave on full power for 60-90 seconds until fully cooked.

4-Seed Rolls

Bread Recipe | **Prep Time:** 1 minute | **Servings:** 1
Per Serving: Kcal: 155, 2.7g Carbs, 8g Protein, 11.1g Fat, 5.9g

Ingredients
- 60g Ground Almonds
- 20g Milled Golden Linseed (Flax)
- 30g Coconut Flour
- 30g Psyllium Husk (whole, blond - not the grey powder)
- 1 tsp Baking Powder
- 200ml Warm Water
- 4 Large Eggs
- 50g Whole Seeds (mixed - we use a bag of sunflower, pumpkin, whole linseed & hemp seeds)
- Salt to taste

Directions
1. Preheat the oven to 180°C.
2. Mix the ground almonds, milled linseed, coconut flour, psyllium husk, baking powder, and salt.
3. Add the warm water and mix.
4. Now add the eggs and whole seeds and mix again. Leave to rest for 5-10 minutes - this will give the coconut flour and psyllium husk time to absorb some moisture.
5. You should now have a dough that holds together when you mold it. Create eight small rolls (use wet hands to stop the mix from sticking) and place them on an oven tray lined with greaseproof baking paper. They won't spread out much, so you don't need to leave lots of space.
6. Bake for 15-20 minutes until golden and firm. Turn the rolls over and bake for 5 minutes to give them a nice crust.
7. Allow cooling slightly before slicing.

90 Second Bread

Bread Recipe | **Prep Time:** 1 minute | **Servings:** 1
Per Serving: Kcal: 296, Carbs (net) 2.8 grams, Protein 14.9 grams, Fat 24.3 grams

Ingredients
- 1 Large Egg
- 35g Ground Almonds or Milled Linseed (or a mix of the two)
- 1/2 tsp Baking Powder
- Seasoning to taste

Directions
1. Mix all of the ingredients in a microwaveable dish. This can be a ramekin, wide mug, or microwavable tub.
2. Microwave on full power for 1 minute. You could also pour the mix onto a panini / George Foreman-style press and cook for a couple of minutes. This makes lovely breadsticks :)

Almond Butter Bread

Bread Recipe | **Prep Time:** 10 minutes | **Servings:** 10
Per Serving: Kcal: 155, Carbs (net) 1 gram, Protein 7.1 grams, Fat 13.1 grams

Ingredients
- 210g Almond Butter (100% almonds)
- 2 Large Eggs
- 8g Chia Seeds
- 5 ml/g Vanilla Extract
- 3g Bicarbonate of Soda
- 25 ml Lemon Juice
- 1/4 tsp Salt

Directions
1. Preheat the oven to 180c.
2. Mix all of the ingredients, except the lemon juice, together until smooth.
3. Add the lemon juice and mix again.
4. Transfer into a lined bread tin - we use a small 9cm x 16cm tin.
5. Bake for around 30 minutes or until firm.

Keto Bara Brith

Bread Recipe | **Prep Time:** 25 minutes | **Servings:** 6
Per Serving: Kcal: 201, 5.3g Carbs, 5.6g Protein, 17.1g Fat

Ingredients
- 100g Boiling water
- 2 Regular Teabags
- 1 Orange zest & Juice (Approx 25g of their juice)
- 30g Mixed fruit
- 100g Ground almonds
- 1/4 tsp Baking powder
- Pinch Salt
- 2 tsp Mixed spice
- 1 large egg
- 50g Melted butter

Directions
1. Oven 170C or 160C in the Ninja grill or the Ninja foodie
2. Brew your tea for 5 minutes, and then remove the tea bags
3. Add your mixed fruit and orange zest. Let it soak in the tea for a minimum of 30 minutes. Overnight is even better but not essential
4. Drain off tea, but keep the fruit and orange zest
5. Add all the dry ingredients to a bowl - Ground almonds, baking powder, and mixed spice and give it a quick mix
6. Now add all the rest of the ingredients, including the soaked mixed fruit and orange zest and 25g of orange juice
7. Mix well
8. Pour all the ingredients into your lined mini loaf tin.
9. Bake for approx 25 minutes, until a skewer popped in the middle, comes out clean
10. Enjoy

Coconut Roti

Bread Recipe | **Prep Time:** 15 minutes | **Servings:** 8
Per Serving: Kcal: 50, Carbs (net) 2.3 grams, Protein 2.5 grams, Fat 1.6 grams

Ingredients
- 100g Coconut Flour
- 20g Psyllium Husks
- 1/2 tsp Baking Powder
- 400ml Warm Water

Directions

1. In a bowl, mix all the dry ingredients. Rub the mix between your fingers to remove any lumps.
2. Add water (the best combination is 1/2 boiled water & 1/2 cold water) and mix with a spoon until it turns into a firm dough - this takes about 30 seconds.
3. Allow the mix to cool for 10-15 minutes.
4. Divide the mix to form 8 dough balls.
5. Place each dough ball between 2 sheets of grease-proof paper and, either using your hands or a rolling pin, create the size and shape roti you want.
6. Heat a good non-stick pan over a medium/high temperature.
7. Peel the roti off the paper and place it in the pan. Cook for 60-90 seconds before turning.
8. Cook the wrap to your taste - the longer you cook it, the crispier it will go. 60-90 seconds on each side will leave it soft.

Dark Linseed Bread

Bread Recipe | **Prep Time:** 15 minutes | **Servings:** 12
Per Serving: Kcal: 89, Carbs (net) 0.7 grams, Protein 4.2 grams, Fat 6.8 grams

Ingredients
- 165g Whole Linseed (golden or brown)
- 50g Sunflower Seeds (or seeds of your choice)
- 3 Large Eggs
- 2 tsp Baking Powder
- 30g Psyllium Husks (the actual husks, not the powder)
- 250ml Luke-Warm Water

Directions
1. Preheat the oven to 160c.
2. Crack the eggs into a large mixing bowl and, using an electric whisk, gradually add the water while mixing at full speed. The eggs should be white and fluffy like a cloud before moving on to the next step.
3. Add all dry ingredients and carefully fold to keep the eggs aerated.
4. Allow the mix to stand for 5 minutes, and it will thicken like a dough.
5. Pour the mix into a lined loaf tin.
6. Bake for 45-60 minutes - times may vary depending on your oven.

Egg Free Bread

Bread Recipe | **Prep Time:** 15 minutes | **Servings:** 12
Per Serving: Kcal: 115, Carbs (net) 2.8 grams, Fat 9.5 grams, Protein 3.7 grams

Ingredients
- 150g Ground Almonds
- 30g Coconut Flour
- 20g Milled Golden Linseed
- 20g Psyllium Husks (the actual husks, not the powder)
- 1/2 tbsp Baking Powder
- 1/4 tsp Salt
- 15ml Olive Oil
- 5ml Apple Cider Vinegar
- 240ml Warm Water

Directions
1. Preheat the oven to 180c.
2. Mix all the dry ingredients in a large mixing bowl.
3. Add the oil and apple cider vinegar and mix well.
4. Add the water and stir.
5. Kneed the mix for 2 - 3 minutes until it creates a dough.
6. Place in a lined loaf tin (we use a small 9 cm x 16 cm tin) and bake for 30 - 35 minutes. Take it out of the container and finish it in the oven for another 10 minutes to give it a better crust.

Family Naan

Bread Recipe | **Prep Time:** 10 minutes | **Servings:** 4
Per Serving: Kcal: 135, 1.8g Carbs, 7.9g Protein, 9.7g Fat

Ingredients
- 80g Milled Linseed
- 2 Large Eggs
- 60ml Warm Water
- 1 tsp Baking Powder
- 1/4 tsp Fast Acting Dried Yeast
- 1/2 tsp Salt
- 1 Garlic Clove, finely chopped (you could replace this with 5g Garlic Puree)
- 1/2 (approx. 5g) Green Chilli, finely chopped
- 10g Fresh Coriander, finely chopped

Directions
1. Preheat the oven to 210°C
2. Mix the linseed with the baking powder, salt, and yeast in a large bowl.
3. Add the eggs and mix to a thick paste.
4. Add the water - mix half boiling and half cold to achieve the correct temperature.
5. Add the chopped garlic, chilli, and coriander to the dough and mix again. This dough will thicken as the linseeds absorb the water.

6. Using wet hands, push the dough out into a 12" baking tray lined with greaseproof paper.
7. Bake for 15 minutes until the bread starts to turn golden brown. Then remove from the oven, turn the bread over, peel the greaseproof paper off, and bake for 5-10 minutes until golden brown on the other side.

Keto Focaccia

Bread Recipe | **Prep Time:** 15 minutes | **Servings:** 8
Per Serving: Kcal: 195, Carbs (net) 3.2 grams, Protein 6.4 grams, Fat 16.5 grams

Ingredients
- 2 tsp Active Dry Yeast (1.5 packets)
- 2 tsp Honey / Sugar (the 'real' stuff)
- 80ml Water (40°C)
- 144g Ground Almonds / Milled Linseed / other milled seeds
- 28g Psyllium Husk
- 1.5 tsp Xanthan Gum
- 1.5 tsp Baking Powder
- 1/2 tsp Salt
- 1 Medium Egg at room temperature
- 2 Med Egg Whites (approx. 60g) at room temperature
- 15ml Olive Oil
- 2 tsp Apple Cider Vinegar
- 2 Sprigs of Rosemary
- 40ml Olive Oil for drizzling & greasing
- Sprinkle of Salt

Directions
1. Set the oven to 50°C (proving temperature).
2. Add the warm water, yeast, and honey to a bowl. Stir it and leave it to foam - this takes about 5-7 minutes.
3. While the yeast is proving, add to another bowl: ground almonds, psyllium husk, xanthan gum, baking powder, and salt, and stir.
4. Once the yeast has started to foam, add the egg, egg whites, olive oil, and vinegar. Mix this all for 2 minutes with a whisk until light and frothy.
5. Add the dry ingredients to the yeast mixture and mix thoroughly until it forms a dough ball.
6. Line a 10" dish (or two smaller dishes - Ella used two 7" trays) with greaseproof paper and grease with 10ml olive oil.
7. Wet your hands (so the dough doesn't stick) and spread the dough across the base of your lined dish.

8. With your wet fingers, make indentations across the dough. Fill some of the indentations with fresh rosemary.
9. Drizzle 30ml olive oil over the top and season.
10. Cover the dish with a tea towel and pop it in the oven to prove for 50 minutes. This dish is not a big riser, but it will look puffy.
11. Pull the dish out of the oven and increase the temperature to 180°C.
12. When the oven is to temperature, return the tray to the oven and cook for 25-30 minutes. Cover the dish with foil after 15 minutes to prevent the top from burning.
13. Allow the bread to cool completely before removing it from the dish.
14. This dish is nice re-toasted before serving :)

Garlic Flatbread

Bread Recipe | **Prep Time:** 15 minutes | **Servings:** 8
Per Serving: Kcal: 134, Carbs (net) 2.1 grams, Protein 7.7 grams, Fat 9.9 grams

Ingredients
- 100g Courgette, grated
- 50g Ground Almonds or Milled Linseed
- 35g Coconut Flour
- 3 Large Eggs
- 60g Grated Mozzarella (we use pre-grated)
- 1 tsp Garlic Powder
- 1 tsp Mixed Herbs
- 1/4 tsp Xanthan Gum
- 1/4 tsp Salt
- Garlic Butter
- 1-2 Garlic Cloves, finely chopped (or 5g Garlic Puree)
- 20g Butter (we like to use salted), melted

Directions
2. Preheat the oven to 180°C.
3. Mix the ground almonds, coconut flour, xanthan gum, and salt.
4. Add the eggs, grated courgette, mozzarella, and mixed herbs. Mix and add any other seasonings/spices at this point.
5. Transfer the mix onto a lined pizza tray. Push the mixture out as far as you can (approx. 10" diameter) and bake for around 20-25 minutes or until golden brown.

6. For the garlic butter, gently heat the butter in a small pan. Add the garlic and fry until the garlic starts to turn nut brown. Add the butter to the baked bread and brush over the top.

Linseed Bread

Bread Recipe | **Prep Time:** 10 minutes | **Servings:** 8
Per Serving: Kcal: 225, Carbs (net) 1.3 grams, Protein 13.5 grams, Fat 17.3 grams

Ingredients
- 250g Milled Golden Linseed (Flax)
- 6 Large Eggs
- 3 tsp Baking Powder
- 180ml Warm Water
- 1 Pack (7g) Fast Acting Dried Yeast

Directions
1. Preheat the oven to 180c.
2. Mix the linseed with the baking powder, a pinch of salt, and the yeast.
3. Add the eggs and mix to a thick paste. It will thicken over time.
4. Add water - mix half boiling and half cold to achieve the correct temperature. If you're making rolls, leave the mix for around 10 minutes - this will allow it to thicken to the point where you can handle the dough.
5. Pour the mix into a lined oven-proof dish or silicone mold. If you're making rolls, use wet hands to form mounds of dough on a tray lined with greaseproof paper. Watch the video at the bottom of this page to see how we do it.
6. Bake for about 45 minutes (or 20-25 minutes for rolls) until it is firm to touch. Times will vary depending on your oven. For a crunchy crust, remove the bread from the greaseproof or mold and pop it back in the range on a baking tray for 5 minutes.

Linseed Wraps

Bread Recipe | **Prep Time:** 10 minutes | **Servings:** 4
Per Serving: Kcal: 170, Carbs (net) 3.4 grams, Protein 5.5 grams, Fat 13.3 grams

Ingredients
- 100g Golden Milled Linseed
- 15g Psyllium Husks
- 1 tbsp Olive Oil
- 1/4 tsp Pink Himalayan Salt
- 250ml Warm Water

Directions

1. Mix the linseed, psyllium husk, salt & oil.
2. Add the water and mix until it becomes a firm dough (around 30 seconds).
3. Allow cooling for 10-15 minutes.
4. Divide the mix into 4 and form a dough ball.
5. Place between 2 sheets of greaseproof paper, and either using your hands or a rolling pin, create the size and shape wrap you want.
6. Use a good non-stick pan over a medium/hot temperature. Peel the wrap off the paper and place it in the pan. Cook for 60-90 seconds before turning.
7. Cook the wrap to your taste - the longer you cook it, the crispier it will go. 60-90 seconds on each side will leave it soft and fluffy.

Mini Naan Breads

Bread Recipe | **Prep Time:** 5 minutes | **Servings:** 4
Per Serving: Kcal: 114, Carbs (net) 1.2 grams, Protein 5.5 grams, Fat 9.4 grams

Ingredients
- 50g Ground Almonds or Milled Linseeds
- 50g Greek or Greek-Style Yogurt
- 1 Large Egg
- 1/2 tsp Baking Powder
- 1 tsp Fresh Coriander Leaf, finely chopped
- 1/2 tsp Cumin Seeds, lightly crushed
- 1/4 tsp Onion or Garlic Powder
- Optional: 1 tsp Nigella Seeds

Directions
1. Add the ground almonds (or milled linseed), baking powder, coriander leaf, cumin seeds, and onion/garlic powder to a mixing bowl.
2. Add the egg and yogurt and mix well until it forms a thick paste.
3. Spoon a quarter of the mix into a good non-stick frying pan over medium/high heat.
4. Cook for 1 minute to allow the mix to firm, and flip over to cook until golden on both sides.
5. Repeat steps 3 & 4 for the rest of the mix.

Parmesan Rolls

Bread Recipe | **Prep Time:** 15 minutes | **Servings:** 6
Per Serving: Kcal: 225, Carbs (net) 2.3 grams, Protein 11.9 grams, Fat 18 grams

Ingredients

- 70g Grated Mozzarella or Mozzarella Block
- 30g Grated Parmesan plus 10g for topping
- 15g Psyllium Husks
- 100g Ground Almonds or other milled nuts/seeds (e.g., sunflower)
- 70g Milled Linseed
- 2 Large Eggs
- 100ml Cold Water
- 1.5 tsp Baking Powder
- 1 tsp Salt
- 1/4 tsp Garlic Powder
- Seasoning of your choice - we used dried mixed herbs

Directions
1. Preheat the oven to 180°C.
2. If you're using a mozzarella block, blitz this in a food processor until it resembles crumbs.
3. Add all the ingredients to 1 big bowl and stir well.
4. Allow the mix to rest for 5-10 minutes.
5. Using wet hands, separate the dough into rolls of equal weight. Place them a few centimeters apart on a lined baking tray.
6. If you're making filled rolls, mix the filling ingredients. Flatten each roll out in the palm of your hand and spoon some of the cream cheese into the center of the dough. Carefully wrap the dough around the filling until it has all been concealed. Repeat for each dough ball and place them back on the tray.
7. Sprinkle the remaining 10g grated parmesan plus the garlic powder and any seasonings on top of the rolls.
8. Bake for 20-25 minutes until firm all around. They will be lovely and crispy on top! If they are going too brown on the outside, knock the temperature down to 160-170°C to ensure they're not doughy in the middle.

Pesto Focaccia

Bread Recipe | **Prep Time:** 15 minutes | **Servings:** 8
Per Serving: Kcal: 168, 1.9g Carbs, 8.4g Protein, 13.5g Fat

Ingredients
- 80g Milled Golden Linseed (Flax)
- 50g Ground Almonds (can be swapped for more linseed or milled sunflower seeds)
- 1 sachet (7g) Fast Acting Dried Yeast
- 1 tsp Baking Powder
- Pinch of Salt
- 3 Large Eggs

- 90ml Warm Water (mix half boiling and half cold)
- 50g Mozzarella (ball or block)
- 30g Pesto (see recipe here)
- 20g Cherry Tomatoes
- Optional: a small handful of seeds to sprinkle on top

Directions

1. Preheat the oven to 170°C.
2. Mix the milled linseed, ground almonds, yeast, baking powder, and salt.
3. Add the eggs and water. Mix again.
4. Pour half of the mix into a 7" or 8" tin (ours is 7" circular), lined with greaseproof baking paper.
5. Break the mozzarella into small chunks and scatter half across the top of the mix in the tin. Then spoon small amounts of pesto on top, using about half.
6. Gently add the remaining linseed mix on top, taking care not to move the mozzarella and pesto too much.
7. Cover the top of the mix with the remaining mozzarella, pesto, and cherry tomatoes, sliced in half. Sprinkle some seeds on top for a nice crunch.
8. Bake for 25-30 minutes, until firm on top. Check the base is fully cooked by gently lifting it out of the tin and making sure the bread comes away from the greaseproof paper as one.
9. Allow to cool slightly, then slice before the mozzarella goes solid. Enjoy!

Tahini Bread

Bread Recipe | **Prep Time:** 5 minutes | **Servings:** 10
Per Serving: Kcal: 160, Carbs (net) 0.6 grams, Protein 7.3 grams, Fat 13.5 grams

Ingredients
- 210g Tahini
- 2 Large Eggs
- 7g Chia Seeds
- 1.5tsp Vanilla Extract
- 1/2 tsp Bicarbonate of Soda
- 1/4 tsp Salt
- 20ml/g Lemon Juice

Directions
1. Preheat the oven to 180°C.
2. Mix all of the ingredients except the lemon juice in a bowl until smooth.
3. Add the lemon juice and mix again. This will react with the bicarbonate of soda, resulting in the mix starting to foam slightly.

4. Transfer the mix to a lined loaf tin. Ours is a mini loaf tin: 9cm x 15cm.
5. Bake for around 30 minutes until firm. The bread will not rise much but should have a good crust round.
6. Nutrition per serving

Zucchini Bread

Bread Recipe | **Prep Time:** 10 minutes | **Servings:** 16
Per Serving: Kcal: 186, Carbs (net) 2.7 grams, Protein 8.3 grams, Fat 15.1 grams

Ingredients
- 150g Grated Courgette
- 5 Large Eggs
- 75g Melted Unsalted Butter, cooled
- 110g Ground Almonds or Milled Linseed
- 70g Coconut Flour
- 100g Grated Mozzarella (not mozzarella ball)
- 1/2 tsp Xanthan Gum
- 1/2 tsp Bicarbonate of Soda
- 2 tsp Baking Powder
- 1/2 tsp Salt
- 1 tsp Dried Oregano

Directions
1. Preheat the oven to 180°C.
2. Whisk the eggs and melted butter together.
3. Mix the ground almonds, coconut flour, xanthan gum, baking powder, baking soda, and salt, and add them to your egg/butter mixture.
4. Add the grated courgette, mozzarella, and oregano. Add any other seasonings and flavours you choose here.
5. Transfer the mix into a lined loaf tin (see the description above for details). For a wide, shallow loaf tin, bake for 1 hour. If you're splitting the mix between two smaller loaf tins, bake for around 40 minutes. The bread should be firm all around.

DRINK RECIPES

Avocado & Raspberry Smoothie

Drink Recipes | **Prep Time:** 5 minutes | **Servings:** 1
Per Serving: Kcal: 137, Carbs (net) 2.5 grams, Protein 2.7 grams, Fat 12.3 grams

Ingredients
- 200ml Unsweetened Almond Milk (or nut-free alternative, e.g., coconut - carton, not tinned)
- 50g Avocado Flesh
- 25g Raspberries (fresh or frozen)
- 1/2 tsp Vanilla Extract or 1/4 tsp Truvia / Natvia / Pure Via Sweetener (adjust to taste)

Directions
1. Use either a Nutri-bullet or jug blender. Pop all of the ingredients in and blitz.
2. Add a dash more milk if the smoothie is very thick because you've used frozen fruit.

Berry & Almond Smoothie

Drink Recipes | **Prep Time:** 5 minutes | **Servings:** 1
Per Serving: Kcal: 171, 4.9g Carbs, 4.1g Protein, 14.8g Fat

Ingredients
- 150ml Unsweetened Almond Milk
- 50g Soft Cream Cheese
- 50g Frozen Berries (we used mixed summer fruit)
- 1/4 tsp Almond Essence
- Truvia / Natvia / Pure Via Sweetener to taste (we added 1/2 tsp)

Directions
1. Add all of the ingredients to a Nutri-bullet / blender and blitz. Adjust the sweetener to taste.

Fat Fuelled Coffee

Made for: Lunch | **Prep Time:** 5 minutes | **Servings:** 1
Per Serving: Kcal: 165, 0g Carbs, 0g Protein, 18.2g Fat

Ingredients
- 1 cup of Black Coffee (can be decaf)
- 10g Unsalted Butter
- 10g Coconut Oil (this can be cooking coconut oil if you're not a fan of the taste)

Directions

1. Make the coffee and pour it into a tall container. Add the butter and coconut oil to the coffee and, using a hand blender, blitz the coffee for 10-15 seconds. This will emulsify the butter and oil, turning the coffee into a latte :)

Hot Chocolate

Drink Recipes | **Prep Time:** 5 minutes | **Servings:** 2
Per Serving: Kcal: 178, Carbs (net) 1.7 grams, Protein 3.4 grams, Fat 16.6 grams

Ingredients
- 450ml Water
- 60ml Unsweetened Almond Milk (or nut-free alternative, e.g., cartooned coconut milk)
- 30g Cocoa Powder
- 50ml Double Cream
- 10g Truvia / Natvia / Pure Via Sweetener
- 2 tsp Vanilla Extract
- Optional: 5g Arrowroot Powder

Directions
2. Whisk the cocoa, sweetener, and 50ml water in a small saucepan over low heat.
3. Add the remaining ingredients and turn the heat up to medium. Whisk occasionally until hot.
4. Taste the mix and add more sweetener if needed.
5. If you're adding arrowroot, mix it with 20ml cold water and stir into the pan.

Kailey's Celtic Butterscotch Cream

Drink Recipes | **Prep Time:** 5 minutes | **Servings:** 2
Per Serving: Kcal: 86, Carbs (net) 0.6 grams, Protein 0.7 grams, Fat 7.7 grams

Ingredients
- 1 Sugar-Free Werther's Original (I know, please don't scoff at the rest of the bag!!! :-
- 30ml Double cream
- 30ml Your favourite milk (I use full-fat Lactose-Free)
- 10ml Whisky

Directions
1. Add to a non-stick saucepan double cream milk and 1 Sugar-free Werther's Original
2. Bring to boil, and immediately turn down to a simmer. Stir until the butterscotch has dissolved. This takes patience :-)
3. Take off the heat, and then add the whisky and mix

4. Divide between 2 shot glasses

Kailey's Celtic Cream

Drink Recipes | **Prep Time:** 5 minutes | **Servings:** 2
Per Serving: Kcal: 163, Carbs (net) 1.1 grams, Protein 1.4 grams, Fat 13.3 grams

Ingredients
- 50ml Double Cream
- 50ml Your favourite Milk (I use Lactose-Free milk)
- 10g Truvia / Natvia / Pure Via Sweetener
- 1/4 tsp Cocoa powder
- 1/4 tsp Vanilla Extract
- 5g coffee granules made up to 10ml boiling water (you decide on how much of this you would like to add. I added half)
- 30ml Whisky

Directions
1. Add all your ingredients (apart from the whisky) to a non-stick saucepan
2. Bring to boil, and turn down to a gentle simmer until the sweetener is dissolved
3. Now add the whisky and mix
4. Pour into 2 shot glasses; I like to add a couple of ice cubes to the mix :-)

Kailey's Celtic Hot Chocolate Cream

Drink Recipes | **Prep Time:** 5 minutes | **Servings:** 2
Per Serving: Kcal: 78, Carbs (net) 2.6 grams, Protein 2.7 grams, Fat 4.8 grams

Ingredients
- 100ml of your favourite milk (I use Lactose-Free milk)
- 5 - 10g Truvia / Natvia / Pure Via Sweetener (Sweeten to taste)
- 5g Cocoa Powder
- 10g 85% Dark Chocolate
- Pinch salt
- Pinch Cinnamon
- Pinch Nutmeg
- 10g Whisky
- Optional extra - Topping of whipped cream, with a grating of dark chocolate

Directions
1. Add all the ingredients to a non-stick saucepan, apart from the whisky and the optional cream topping
2. Bring to boil and turn down to a gentle simmer, stirring continuously until all the ingredients are combined
3. Now stir in the whisky and gently heat through

4. Pour into 2 glasses
5. Optional extra whipped cream, approx 15 to 20g per glass, with some grated chocolate on top

Kailey's Celtic Non-Alcoholic Cream

Drink Recipes | **Prep Time:** 5 minutes | **Servings:** 2
Per Serving: Kcal: 132, Carbs (net) 0.4 grams, Protein 0.4 grams, Fat 14.3 grams

Ingredients
- A glass/mug of your favourite black coffee
- 30ml Double Cream
- 5-10g Truvia / Natvia / Pure Via Sweetener or sweeten to taste
- 1/4 tsp Vanilla Extract
- Pinch Cinnamon
- Pinch Nutmeg
- Pinch Ginger
- 30ml Whisked Double Cream

Directions
1. Add to a non-stick saucepan, double cream (not the whisked up cream), and sweetener
2. Bring to boil, and immediately turn down to a simmer. Stir until the sweetener has dissolved.
3. Take off the heat, and add all the other ingredients (apart from the coffee & whipped cream).
4. Now make your favourite black coffee
5. Add the whipped cream to the cooling cream mixture and gently mix well
6. Finally, stir the coffee well until it's spinning, and gently pour 1/2 of the cream mixture close to the top of the coffee. If you do it like this, the cream mixture should float on the top

Peanut Butter & Cocoa Milkshake

Drink Recipes | **Prep Time:** 5 minutes | **Servings:** 1
Per Serving: Kcal: 175, 4.5g Carbs, 7.9g Protein, 13.6g Fat

Ingredients
- 150ml Unsweetened Almond Milk (see alternatives below)
- 30g Greek / Greek-style Yogurt
- 15g Peanut Butter (100% nuts)
- 5g Cocoa Powder
- Truvia / Natvia / Pure Via Sweetener to taste (we added 1/2 tsp)

Directions
1. Add all of the ingredients to a Nutri-bullet / blender and blitz. Adjust the sweetener to taste.

SWEET TREAT RECIPES

Almond Cake

Sweet Treat Recipe | **Prep Time:** 15 minutes | **Servings:** 6
Per Serving: Kcal: 192, Carbs (net) 1.3 grams, Protein 5.6 grams, Fat 18.4 grams

Ingredients
- 150ml Olive Oil
- 3 Large Eggs
- 3 tsp Almond Extract
- 250g Ground Almonds
- 50-60g Truvia / Natvia / Pure Via Sweetener
- 1/2 tsp Bicarbonate of Soda
- Pinch of salt

Directions
1. Preheat the oven to 170°C (reduce this to 150°C if you use a fan oven).
2. Add the olive oil, eggs, and almond extract to a Nutri-bullet blender. Blend for a few seconds until it forms a runny mayonnaise.
3. Mix the dry ingredients in a bowl.
4. Add the egg & oil mixture to the dry ingredients and mix until thoroughly combined.
5. Line an 8" brownie tin with greaseproof paper and pour in your cake mix.
6. Bake for around 40 minutes until firm.

Baking in the Ninja Foodi
1. I split the mix into two and bake in a small loaf tin (only one fits in the Ninja at a time). Alternatively, line a round cake tin (7-8").
2. Use the Bake function at 150°C. Bake for 25-30minutes, checking at the 25-minute mark to see if it's firm.

Avocado Brownies

Sweet Treat Recipe | **Prep Time:** 15 minutes | **Servings:** 16
Per Serving: Kcal: 140, Carbs (net) 3.6 grams, Protein 3.6 grams, Fat 12.1 grams

Ingredients
- 250g Avocado Flesh
- 40g Cocoa Powder
- 90g Ground Almonds
- 35g Coconut Oil
- 100g 85% Dark Chocolate
- 40g Truvia / Natvia / Pure Via Sweetener
- 1/2 tsp Vanilla Extract
- 2 Large Eggs (see the description for alternative)

Directions
1. Preheat the oven to 190°C.
2. Melt the dark chocolate and coconut oil in a bowl over a pan of boiling water or in the microwave. If using a pan, make sure that no water gets into the chocolate mixture. Allow cooling slightly.
3. Using a food processor, blend the avocado until smooth.
4. Add the eggs, vanilla extract, and cocoa powder. Process again until smooth.
5. Gradually add the melted chocolate/oil mix while the food processor is on to mix the ingredients.
6. Finally, add the ground almonds and sweetener and blend. The mixture should resemble a thick mousse.
7. Spread the mix into a square 8" tin lined with greaseproof paper. Bake for 20-25 minutes. If you want the brownies extra gooey, reduce the cooking time slightly.
8. Allow the brownies to cool before cooking as they're quite fragile fully. They firm up once they're in the fridge.

Berry Tray Bake

Sweet Treat Recipe | **Prep Time:** 15 minutes | **Servings:** 16
Per Serving: Kcal: 103, Carbs (net) 2 grams, Protein 3.5 grams, Fat 8.6 grams

Ingredients
- 75g Butter
- 55g Ground Almonds (or other milled nuts/seeds, e.g., milled linseed)
- 35g Coconut Flour
- 50g Grated Mozzarella
- 1/4 tsp Xanthan Gum
- 1/4 tsp Bicarbonate of Soda
- 1 tsp Baking Powder
- 25g Desiccated Coconut
- 3 Large Eggs
- 1.5 tsp Vanilla Essence
- 30g Truvia / Natvia / Pure Via Sweetener (add more to taste)
- 150g Mixed Berries

Directions
1. Preheat the oven to 180°C.
2. Melt the butter and allow it to cool slightly.
3. Mix all of the dry ingredients in a bowl.
4. In a separate bowl, whisk up the eggs and then whisk in the cooled, melted butter and vanilla extract.
5. Add the mozzarella, frozen berries, and dry ingredients to the egg/butter mix. Gently combine these with a spatula.

6. Transfer the mixture to a lined tin and bake for around 30-40 minutes until firm.

Keto Bethmannchen

Sweet Treat Recipe | **Prep Time:** 15 minutes | **Servings:** 16
Per Serving: Kcal: 41, Carbs (net) 0.4 grams, Protein 1.7 grams, Fat 3.5 grams

Ingredients
- 300g Ground Almonds (or other milled nuts/seeds)
- 60g Truvia / Natvia / Pure Via Sweetener
- 2 Medium Egg Yolks
- 1 tsp Almond Essence (omit this or swap it for vanilla extract if you're not a fan of marzipan)
- 40 - 60ml Water
- One flaked Almond per biscuit

Directions
2. Preheat the oven to 200°C
3. Place all of the ingredients in a bowl and beat them all together until it forms a dough
4. Taking a small pinch of the dough at a time, form tiny spheres and place them on a lined baking tray
5. Press a flaked almond into the top of each sphere to create a little dent
6. Bake for about 20 - 25 minutes, until slightly crispy. They will crisp more as they cool. Keep an eye on them from about 15 minutes onwards to make sure that they don't burn

Blackcurrant Muffins

Sweet Treat Recipe | **Prep Time:** 15 minutes | **Servings:** 8
Per Serving: Kcal: 125, Carbs (net) 2.8 grams, Protein 6 grams, Fat 8.9 grams

Ingredients
- 50g Softened Cream Cheese
- 25g Truvia / Natvia / Pure Via Sweetener
- 3 Large Eggs
- 30ml Unsweetened Almond Milk
- 40g Ground Almonds
- 40g Coconut Flour
- 2 tsp Lemon Juice
- 1 tsp Vanilla Extract
- 1 tsp Baking Powder
- 60g Frozen Blackcurrants (keep these in the freezer right up until you add them to the mix)
- 30g Flaked Almonds

Directions

1. Preheat the oven to 180°C.
2. Use an electric whisk to mix the cream cheese and sweetener.
3. Add the eggs and almond milk and whisk again.
4. Add the remaining ingredients, except the fruit, and mix until smooth.
5. The fruit needs to be straight from the freezer so add these last. Gently combine with the rest of the ingredients.
6. Pour the cake mix into silicone muffin cases and sprinkle the flaked almonds on top.
7. Bake for 15-20 minutes until firm.

Black Forest Gateau

Sweet Treat Recipe | **Prep Time:** 10 minutes | **Servings:** 4
Per Serving: Kcal: 183, Carbs (net) 4.7 grams, Protein 3.1 grams, Fat 16.4 grams

Ingredients
- 100g Cooked Mixed Berries or Homemade Jam
- 30g 85% Dark Chocolate
- 1 Egg
- 1 tsp Truvia / Natvia / Pure Via Sweetener
- 95g Double Cream
- 1 tsp Vanilla Extract
- 1/4 tsp Baking Powder
- Pinch of salt

Directions
1. Melt the chocolate in the microwave for 30 seconds to ensure it doesn't burn.
2. Meanwhile, whisk 80g of cream until soft peaks form and set aside.
3. Whisk 1 egg in a bowl and put it to one side.
4. In a separate bowl, add 20g melted chocolate, the sweetener, whisked egg, vanilla extract, baking powder, salt, and the remaining 15g un-whisked cream. Mix and microwave for 1 minute (this cake doesn't need to look perfect in shape.
5. Divide the cooked berries between each pot.
6. Break the cake into pieces and add a quarter to each pot.
7. Add 20g whipped cream to each pot and drizzle melted chocolate over the top.

Chocolate Brownies

Sweet Treat Recipe | **Prep Time:** 10 minutes | **Servings:** 16
Per Serving: Kcal: 136, Carbs (net) 1.8 grams, Protein 3 grams, Fat 12.6 grams

Ingredients

- 100g 85% Dark Chocolate
- 80g Unsalted Butter
- 60g Double Cream
- 3 Large Eggs (for nut-free brownies, increase this to 4 eggs)
- 70g Ground Almonds (for nut-free, swap the ground almonds for 25g Coconut Flour)
- 30g Truvia / Natvia / Pure Via Sweetener
- 1 tsp Baking Powder
- 1 tsp Vanilla Extract
- 20g Cocoa Powder

Directions

1. Preheat the oven to 180°C.
2. Melt the butter and chocolate in the microwave or over a pot of boiling water (make sure no water gets into the chocolate).
3. Add the cream to the melted chocolate/butter and stir. This will cool the mixdown.
4. Add the remaining ingredients and mix until smooth.
5. Line an 8" square tray with greaseproof baking paper and pour the mix in. Evenly spread it in the tin.
6. Bake for around 15 minutes. the top should be just firm to touch - if you bake them for less time, you'll have super gooey brownies :D
7. Allow to cool a little and then cut into squares.

Butterscotch Pudding

Sweet Treat Recipe | **Prep Time:** 5 minutes | **Servings:** 2
Per Serving: Kcal: 247, Carbs (net) 1.1 grams, Protein 2.2 grams, Fat 26.1 grams

Ingredients

- 100 g Fresh Double Cream
- 5 Sugar-Free Werther's Original (the hard-boiled ones, not the chewy ones)
- 1 Egg Yolk

Directions

1. Heat the cream and the Butterscotch Werthers until the sweets have melted, and allow to cool slightly.
2. Beat in the egg yolk.
3. Return to heat and cook gently for about 3 minutes, stirring continuously.
4. Divide between 2 small pudding pots (I used shot glasses).

Butterscotch Sauce

Sweet Treat Recipe | **Prep Time:** 5 minutes | **Servings:** 4
Per Serving: Kcal: 88, 0.3g Carbs, 0.3g Protein, 9.5g Fat

Ingredients

Original Version

- 80g Fresh Double Cream
- 6 Sugar-Free Werthers Original (the hard-boiled ones, not the chewy ones)

Cleaner Version

- 100ml Unsweetened Almond Milk
- 30g Unsalted Butter
- 30g Double Cream
- 10g Truvia / Natvia / Pure Via Sweetener (adjust to taste)
- 1 tsp Vanilla Extract or Toffee Flavdrops from MyProtein

Directions

Original Version

1. Put the cream and butterscotch sweets into a nonstick saucepan.
2. Gently melt while stirring constantly. This will thicken into a thick glossy sauce (this takes about 5 minutes)

Cleaner Version

1. Add all of the ingredients to a nonstick saucepan.
2. Gently heat, stirring to melt the butter. Allow it to bubble and reduce on medium heat, stirring occasionally. You will notice the sauce gets gradually thicker.
3. After 10-15 minutes, the sauce thickened quite a bit. Allow it to rest for a couple of minutes - it will start to separate slightly. Mix this back together to form a glossy sauce.

Caramel Clusters

Sweet Treat Recipe | **Prep Time:** 15 minutes | **Servings:** 20
Per Serving: Kcal: 124, Carbs (net) 0.8 grams, Protein 1.2 grams, Fat 12.6 grams

Ingredients

- 60g Unsalted Butter
- 90g Double Cream
- 20g Truvia / Natvia / Pure Via Sweetener
- 200g Crushed Nuts (we like to use pecans) - either blitz these in a food processor or crush them by hand, e.g., in a pestle & mortar
- 50g 85% Dark Chocolate

Directions

1. In a medium-sized pan that you can whisk in, melt the butter. Allow it to turn golden brown. There's no need to stir it at this point.
2. Reduce the heat and add the cream while whisking. Whisk for 20-30 seconds, and then add the sweetener.
3. Turn the heat back up, continue to whisk, and allow it to come to boil - this will bubble and thicken, turning golden brown. This process will only take 3-4 minutes from start to finish.
4. Add the crushed nuts to the caramel and stir to coat them.
5. Divide the mix into little silicone molds or ice cube trays. Put them in the freezer to set for around 10 minutes.
6. While the clutters are setting, melt the chocolate and allow it to cool slightly.
7. Drizzle the chocolate over the clusters.
8. Place them back in the fridge or freezer to set.

Choc Chip Cookies

Sweet Treat Recipe | **Prep Time:** 15 minutes | **Servings:** 15
Per Serving: Kcal: 122, Carbs (net) 1.2 grams, Protein 2.4 grams, Fat 11.8 grams

Ingredients
- 100g Unsalted Butter
- 1 tsp Vanilla Extract
- 115g Ground Almonds
- 30-40g Truvia / Natvia / Pure Via Sweetener
- 1/2 tsp Baking Powder
- 1/2 tsp Xanthan Gum
- 1 Large Egg
- 50g 85% Dark Chocolate

Directions
1. Preheat the oven to 180°C.
2. Melt the butter in the microwave or over a pot of boiling water.
3. Add the sweetener and vanilla extract and whisk.
4. Add the ground almonds, sweetener, baking powder, and xanthan gum mix, and add the egg. Mix again.
5. Chop the dark chocolate into chips and combine. Or, for crispier cookies, leave the chocolate aside for later.
6. Line a tray with greaseproof baking paper or use a silicone tray.

7. Using wet hands, separate the mix and press the cookies into shape. They won't spread out in the oven so press them out into the shape you'd like them. For crispier cookies, press them out as flat as possible.
8. Bake for 15 minutes or until golden. You may want to flip them over to allow them to go golden on both sides. Be careful; they're quite squishy when they first come out of the oven!
9. Allow cooling fully. For the crispier cookies, melt the chocolate and spread a layer (or delicately drizzle) over the top of the cookies.

Chocolate Fudge Truffles

Sweet Treat Recipe | **Prep Time:** 15 minutes | **Servings:** 15
Per Serving: Kcal: 57, Carbs (net) 1.1 grams, Protein 0.9 grams, Fat 5.2 grams

Ingredients
- 100g Avocado Flesh (over-ripe is best)
- 50g 85% Dark Chocolate
- 15g Coconut Oil (we use cooking coconut oil which has no taste or smell)
- 20g Cocoa Powder
- 25g Truvia / Natvia / Pure Via Sweetener
- 1/2 tsp Vanilla Extract (plus any additional flavorings, e.g., orange essence)
- 20g Crushed Pecans or Hazelnuts (or other nuts - I blitz these in the Nutri-bullet for just a second or two)

Directions
1. Melt the chocolate and coconut oil in the microwave (in 30-second bursts) or over a pot of boiling water.
2. Roughly chop the avocado, add it to a small food processor and blitz it into small chunks.
3. Add the melted chocolate and oil to the avocado and blitz again. You may need to use a spoon to scrape some mix off the sides of the processor to allow it to combine fully.
4. Add all remaining ingredients (except the crushed nuts) and blitz for a final time. Taste the mix and adjust the flavorings at this point.
5. Pour the crushed nuts into a small bowl.
6. Take a small chunk of the mix (around 10g) and gently roll it into a truffle with your hands. Place the truffle in the crushed nuts and shake until fully coated. Repeat until all of the mixes have been used up.

7. I like to store these in the freezer, and I'm not tempted to eat one every time I open the fridge!

Chocolate Lava Cake

Sweet Treat Recipe | **Prep Time:** 15 minutes | **Servings:** 15
Per Serving: Kcal: 217, Carbs (net) 2.4 grams, Protein 10.5 grams, Fat 17.1 grams

Ingredients
- 20g Cocoa Powder
- 10g Truvia / Natvia / Pure Via Sweetener
- 1 Large Egg
- 15ml Fresh Double Cream or Almond Milk
- 1/2 tsp Vanilla Extract
- 1/4 tsp Baking Powder
- A pinch of salt
- Optional: 1 heaped tsp Instant Coffee

Directions
1. Mix all of the ingredients in a microwavable / oven-proof bowl.
2. Microwave on full power for 50-60 seconds, or bake at 180c for 10-15 minutes. The cake should be firm on top but should still be gooey in the middle :)

Chocolate & Orange Marmalade Cake

Sweet Treat Recipe | **Prep Time:** 15 minutes | **Servings:** 8
Per Serving: Kcal: 259, Carbs (net) 5.6 grams, Protein 7.5 grams, Fat 22.1 grams

Ingredients
- 100g Soft Cream Cheese
- 60g Softened Unsalted Butter
- 60ml/g Unsweetened Almond Milk
- 3 Large Eggs
- 130g Ground Almonds
- 30g Truvia / Natvia / Pure Via Sweetener
- 20g Coconut Flour
- 2 tsp Lemon Juice
- 1 tsp Vanilla Extract
- 1 tsp Baking Powder
- 80g Homemade Orange Marmalade
- 25g 85% Dark Chocolate

Directions
1. If you haven't done so already, make the marmalade using the recipe here.
2. Preheat the oven to 180°C.
3. Add the cream cheese and butter to a bowl. Whisk until soft peaks form. We use an electric whisk.
4. Add the almond milk and eggs and mix again - don't have the whisk on a high setting!

5. Add the ground almonds, sweetener, coconut flour, lemon juice, vanilla extract, and baking powder.
6. Mix everything and then pour the cake batter into a lined 8" tin (spring-form is best).
7. Gently add the marmalade all over the top of the batter - you don't want this to sink too far into the cake mix.
8. Bake for around 35 minutes until golden and firm to touch.
9. Once cooked, allow the cake to cool slightly in the tins before removing it and placing it on a cooling rack.
10. Melt the chocolate and use a spoon to drizzle it on top of the cake - I don't like to completely cover it in chocolate because the marmalade topping looks too pretty!

Chocolate & Raspberry Ice Cream

Sweet Treat Recipe | **Prep Time:** 5 minutes | **Servings:** 8
Per Serving: Kcal: 204, 2.8g Carbs, 2.4g Protein, 19.4g Fat

Ingredients
- 150g Avocado Flesh
- 120g Tinned Coconut Milk (as high % coconut as you can find - Lidl seems to be best for this)
- 120g Double Cream or more Tinned Coconut Milk
- 30g Truvia / Natvia / Pure Via Sweetener
- 40g Cocoa Powder
- 100g Raspberries (fresh or frozen) - sub for any other berries but raspberries work the best!
- 2 tsp Vanilla Extract
- Optional: 25g 85% Dark Chocolate, chopped into small pieces (add these once everything has been blitzed together)

Directions
1. Place all of the ingredients in a food processor and blend until smooth. We add the raspberries afterward to keep them whole.
2. Place in the freezer to set. If it's been in the freezer for a while, take it out to defrost slightly before scooping.

Choco Waffles

Sweet Treat Recipe | **Prep Time:** 5 minutes | **Servings:** 4

Per Serving: Kcal: 156, Carbs (net) 2.9 grams, Protein 11.2 grams, Fat 8.9 grams

Ingredients
- 4 Large Eggs
- 80ml Unsweetened Almond Milk (or other milk of your choice - e.g., cartooned coconut 'milk')
- 35g Coconut Flour
- 10g Cocoa Powder
- 25g Truvia / Natvia / Pure Via Sweetener
- 1 tsp Vanilla Essence / Extract
- 1/2 tsp Baking Powder

Directions
1. Whisk the eggs, milk, and vanilla together in a bowl.
2. Add the remaining ingredients and whisk until smooth.
3. Pour a third of the mix in a good non-stick pan, a crepe pan, or a waffle press. If you're cooking these in a pan, you may need to add around 5g of butter to the pan first and pour the mix into smaller amounts to make lots of mini pancakes instead of a few large ones. Allow the mix to cool until air bubbles appear on the top. Gently turn the pancake over to finish cooking. If you open your waffle press too early, the waffle may split in half!

Cinnamon Crunch

Sweet Treat Recipe | **Prep Time:** 5 minutes | **Servings:** 10
Per Serving: Kcal: 97, Carbs (net) 1.7 grams, Protein 2.1 grams, Fat 8.7 grams

Ingredients
- 25g Unsalted Butter or Coconut Oil (Cooking Coconut Oil has no taste)
- 50g Coconut Chips / Flakes
- 30g Sunflower Seeds
- 30g Pumpkin Seeds
- 20g Whole Golden Linseed
- 10-15g Truvia / Natvia / Pure Via Sweetener
- 1/2 tsp Vanilla Extract
- 1/2 - 1 tsp Mixed Spice or Cinnamon (adjust to taste)

Directions
1. Preheat the oven to 180°C.
2. Melt the butter/coconut oil in the microwave or a small saucepan over gentle heat.

3. Add the melted butter/oil to a mixing bowl and all other ingredients and mix well to coat the seeds & coconut chips with the spice & sweetener. Adjust the sweetener to taste - we use very little as the coconut chips are quite sweet.
4. Transfer the mix to an oven tray (if it's not very non-stick, line it with greaseproof baking paper or a silicone mat) and bake for around 10-15 minutes until golden. You may need to stir the mix halfway through baking to prevent the sides from burning.
5. Allow cooling before transferring to a storage container/jar. Keep in a cool cupboard (it'll last several weeks... although we eat it too quickly!).

Classic Vanilla Muffins

Sweet Treat Recipe | **Prep Time:** 10minutes | **Servings:** 12
Per Serving: Kcal: 128, Carbs (net) 0.8 grams, Protein 3.8 grams, Fat 11.9 grams

Ingredients
- 120g Double Cream or Tinned Coconut Milk (as high % coconut as you can find)
- 2 Large Eggs
- 1 tsp Vanilla Extract
- 130g Ground Almonds
- 30g Truvia / Natvia / Pure Via Sweetener
- 1 tsp Baking Powder
- Pinch of salt
- Optional: 25g 85% Dark Chocolate, chopped into small pieces

Directions
1. Preheat the oven to 180°C.
2. In a large bowl, add the cream. Eggs and vanilla extract and mix.
3. Add the remaining ingredients and mix again. Taste and adjust the sweetness if necessary.
4. Divide the mix into silicone cupcake cases.
5. Bake for 15-20 minutes or until golden.

Coconut Macaroons

Sweet Treat Recipe | **Prep Time:** 10 minutes | **Servings:** 15
Per Serving: Kcal: 131, Carbs (net) 2.4 grams, Protein 1.6 grams, Fat 12.8 grams

Ingredients
- 200g Unsweetened Desiccated Coconut (check the label, it should be around 6g carbs per 100g)

- 200g Full Fat Tinned Coconut Milk (check the label, you want a high coconut extract %. Around 70% coconut is good)
- 1 tsp Vanilla Extract
- 1 Large Egg White
- 50-75g Homemade Jam
- 50g 85% Dark Chocolate

Directions
1. Preheat the oven to 180°C.
2. Mix the desiccated coconut, coconut milk, and vanilla extract in a large bowl.
3. In a separate bowl, whisk the white of a large egg using an electric whisk to form light fluffy peaks.
4. Fold the egg white into the coconut mix.
5. Line a baking tray with baking paper and divide the coconut mix into 15 equal portions. Press the mix with the back of a spoon to compact the macaroon.
6. Add a little dollop of jam to the top of each macaroon.
7. Bake for 12-15 minutes or until golden brown.
8. Allow to cool on the tray, and then put the tray in the fridge for 30 minutes. This will allow the macaroons to the firm.
9. Melt the dark chocolate and either drizzle across the top or turn the macaroons over and spoon a little dark chocolate on the base.
10. Pop back in the fridge to allow the chocolate to set.

Coconut Vanilla Muffins

Sweet Treat Recipe | **Prep Time:** 10 minutes | **Servings:** 12
Per Serving: Kcal: 85, Carbs (net) 0.8 grams, Protein 2.6 grams, Fat 7.6 grams

Ingredients
- 3 Large Eggs
- 130ml Double Cream or Tinned Coconut Milk (as high % coconut as you can find - we've found that Lidl is best for this)
- 40g Coconut Flour
- 30g Truvia / Natvia / Pure Via Sweetener
- 1 tsp Baking Powder
- 1 tsp Vanilla Extract
- Optional: 25g 85% Dark Chocolate, chopped into tiny pieces

Directions
1. Preheat the oven to 180°C.
2. In a large bowl, add the cream. Eggs and vanilla extract and mix.
3. Add the remaining ingredients and mix again. Taste and adjust the sweetness if necessary.

4. Divide the mix into silicone cupcake cases.
5. Bake for 15-20 minutes or until golden.

Coffee Cake

Sweet Treat Recipe | **Prep Time:** 15 minutes | **Servings:** 12
Per Serving: Kcal: 156, 1.6g Carbs, 3.2g Protein, 14.5g Fat

Ingredients

Cake
- 180g Double Cream
- 3 Large Eggs (use 4 large eggs if using coconut flour instead of almonds)
- 1.5 tsp Vanilla Extract
- 195g Ground Almonds (or replace this with 50g Coconut Flour)
- 45g Truvia / Natvia / Pure Via Sweetener
- 5g Instant Coffee (adjust to taste)
- 1.5 tsp Baking Powder
- Pinch of salt

For the cream:
- 100g Double Cream
- 1 tsp Vanilla Extract
- Sweetener if needed (you could blitz this to a powder in a Nutribullet style blender if you prefer)

Directions
1. Preheat the oven to 180°C.
2. Add the cream, eggs, and vanilla extract and whisk in a large bowl.
3. Add the ground almonds (or coconut flour), sweetener, instant coffee granules, baking powder, and salt. Combine with the egg mix until smooth. If you're using coconut flour, don't be alarmed if it looks very runny - it thickens as the coconut flour absorbs some of the liquid.
4. Pour into a lined 8" tin and bake for 25-30 minutes or until just firm on top.
5. Allow the cake to cool fully while you make the topping.
6. Add the cream and vanilla extract into a bowl and whisk until soft peaks form (we use an electric whisk here). Add sweetener if required.
7. Either cut the cake in half, fill it with cream, or add the cream on top once it's completely cooled.

Cookie Dough Fat Bombs

Sweet Treat Recipe | **Prep Time:** 10 minutes | **Servings:** 15
Per Serving: Kcal: 122, Carbs (net) 1.6 grams, Protein 4.3 grams, Fat 10.4 grams

Ingredients
- 100g Almond Butter (100% nuts)
- 150g Ground Almonds (or other milled nuts/seeds)
- 20g Coconut Flour
- 100ml Unsweetened Almond Milk
- 25g 85% Dark Chocolate
- 10g Truvia / Natvia / Pure Via Sweetener
- 2 tsp Vanilla Extract

Directions
1. Mix the almond butter, ground almond and coconut flour. If you're using crunchy almond butter, you may find it easier to heat this in the microwave to help with mixing it in quickly.
2. Add the rest of the ingredients and combine fully. Sweeten to taste.
3. Using wet hands, roll pieces of dough between your palms to form a ball.
4. Place in the fridge for doughy bites or the freezer for a more solid treat.

Pancakes (Crepes)

Sweet Treat Recipe | **Prep Time:** 1 minute | **Servings:** 4
Per Serving: Kcal: 147, Carbs (net) 7.1 grams, Fat 11.2 grams, Protein 3.7 grams

Ingredients
- 60ml Double Cream
- 60ml Your favourite milk (I used Full fat Lactose-Free)
- 2 eggs
- 15g Arrowroot Powder
- Sweeten to taste - optional (leave the sweetener out for a savoury crepe)

Directions
1. Put all the ingredients in a food blender or a bowl and whisk till smooth
2. Get your suitable nonstick pan hot, with a little oil if needed
3. Pour a quarter into your pan and carefully spread it out thin
4. Cook for approx 30 - 60 seconds
5. Flip over and do the same on the other side

Keto Custard

Sweet Treat Recipe | **Prep Time:** 5 minutes | **Servings:** 6
Per Serving: Kcal: 186, Carbs (net) 0.9 grams, Protein 1.4 grams, Fat 19.5 grams

Ingredients
- 200ml/g Double Cream
- 2 Large Egg Yolks
- 1 tsp Vanilla Extract or 1/2 tsp Vanilla Bean Paste
- 5g Truvia / Natvia / Pure Via Sweetener (adjust to taste)

Directions
1. Heat the cream over low heat in a small non-stick frying pan until it starts to bubble gently.
2. Remove from heat and add the vanilla and egg yolks while gently whisking.
3. As the eggs fully combine, return the pan to the heat and allow it to come back to a boil.
4. Keep the custard moving at all times, and if it starts to stick to the bottom of the pan, remove it from heat.

Festive Apple Crunch

Sweet Treat Recipe | **Prep Time:** 5 minutes | **Servings:** 6
Per Serving: Kcal: 256, 6.8g Carbs, 4.9g Protein, 22.6g Fat

Ingredients
- 300g Cooking Apple - Peeled, cored & chunkily chopped
- 150g Mixed nuts (we used pecans, hazelnuts & flaked almonds) - chunky chop by hand - do not blitz in the food processor
- 60g Melted butter
- 1 tsp Vanilla extract
- 1/2 tsp Ground cinnamon or Mixed Spice
- 20g Truvia / Natvia / Pure Via Sweetener

Directions
1. Preheat the oven to 190°C (or Ninja to 180°C).
2. Add all your ingredients to a bowl and mix well.
3. If you need to adjust the sweetener, Taste the mix, then spread it evenly across an oven dish.
4. Bake for 25-30 minutes.
5. As a cake topping...
6. Make a vanilla sponge mix using the Classic Vanilla Cake recipe in a 7" spring-form tin, and before baking, sprinkle on some Festive Apple Crunch to cover the top of the cake. Then bake until the cake has set.

Keto Granola

Sweet Treat Recipe | **Prep Time:** 10 minutes | **Servings:** 12
Per Serving: Kcal: 105, Carbs (net) 0.8 grams, Protein 2.2 grams, Fat 10.1 grams

Ingredients

- 100g Nuts of your choice (e.g., Almonds, Pecans, Brazil Nuts, Hazelnuts)
- 45g Milled Linseed (or other milled nuts/seeds)
- 15g Flaked Almonds
- 25g Coconut Oil or Unsalted Butter
- 20g Truvia / Natvia / Pure Via Sweetener

Directions

1. Preheat the oven to 180°C.
2. Roughly chop the nuts of your choice (except the flaked almonds) in a food processor or by hand. You still want some chunks to give the granola a crunch.
3. Add the nuts to a mixing bowl and the seeds, flaked almonds, and sweeteners.
4. Melt the coconut oil or butter in the microwave and add this to your dry ingredients. Mix to coat the nuts and seeds in the oil.
5. Spread the granola mixture onto a baking tray lined with greaseproof paper (or a silicone mat) and bake for about 10 minutes or until golden brown. Be careful - they'll burn quickly!

Granola Bars

Sweet Treat Recipe | **Prep Time:** 10 minutes | **Servings:** 8
Per Serving: Kcal: 163, Carbs (net) 2.2 grams, Protein 4.2 grams, Fat 14.9 grams

Ingredients

- 100g Nuts of your choice (almonds, pecans, brazil, hazelnuts) - we prefer flaked almonds, whole pecans, and whole hazelnuts.
- 60g Milled Linseed
- 25g Coconut Oil or Butter
- 1 Large Egg
- 30g Truvia / Natvia / Pure Via Sweetener
- 25g 85% Dark Chocolate

Directions

1. Preheat the oven to 180°C.
2. Chop the nuts of your choice in a food processor. You still want some chunks to give the bars more of a crunch. We would add whole almonds, hazelnuts, or brazil nuts before pecans, as the latter takes less time to break down. We don't add flaked almonds to the processor as we prefer to leave them as they are :)
3. Transfer the nuts to a mixing bowl. Add the linseeds and sweetener and mix.

4. Melt the coconut oil or butter and add this to the mixing bowl, coating the nuts & seeds.
5. Crack the egg into the bowl and combine it with the rest of the mixture.
6. Press the mixture into a lined oven mixture (we use around a 7" tray) and bake for around 15 minutes or until golden brown. Depending on your oven, you may want to flip them over to brown on both sides.
7. Melt the dark chocolate and drizzle on top of your baked granola bars.
8. Allow the chocolate to solidify before cutting - the solid chocolate helps to reduce crumbs when chopping up.

Jaffa Cakes

Sweet Treat Recipe | **Prep Time:** 15 minutes | **Servings:** 12
Per Serving: Kcal: 78, Carbs (net) 1.9 grams, Protein 3.1 grams, Fat 6 grams

Ingredients

- 1 Packet of Orange Hartley's Sugar-Free Jelly Powder (other flavours, like raspberry, also work nicely)
- 110ml Boiling Water
- 2 Eggs
- 30g Truvia / Natvia / Pure Via Sweetener
- 1 tsp Orange Essence (optional) makes it a bit more orange zingy, but not essential!
- 45g Almond Butter
- 15g Coconut Flour
- 70g 85% Dark Chocolate

Directions

1. Preheat the oven to 180°C.
2. Boil the kettle and pour 110ml into a small jug.
3. Add the sugar-free jelly powder to the water and quickly stir until it's all dissolved.
4. Pour into mini cake molds, preferably smaller than the molds you're using for the bases.
5. Pop in the fridge until they have set - usually at least 45 minutes.
6. Whisk together the eggs, orange essence (if you're using it), and sweetener until pale in color and airy.
7. Add the almond butter and coconut flour. Fold them into the egg mix with a spatula.
8. Divide the mix across silicone cake molds and flatten it down.

9. Cook for about 12 minutes until slightly golden.
10. Allow the bases to cool fully. When the jelly is set, top the cakes with the jelly.
11. Meanwhile, melt the chocolate in the microwave in 30-second bursts.
12. Allow the chocolate to cool, and then carefully drizzle it over the jelly and base. Allow the chocolate to set.

Ketobix

Sweet Treat Recipe | **Prep Time:** 10 minutes | **Servings:** 24
Per Serving: Kcal: 65, 0.6g Carbs, 1.3g Protein, 6g Fat

Ingredients
- 50g Mixed Nuts
- 50g Mixed Seeds
- 50g POTATO FIBRE
- Pinch Salt
- 20g Ground Chia seeds
- 10g Truvia / Natvia / Pure Via Sweetener

- 100g Melted butter
- 100ml Water

Directions
1. Oven 120C, Ninja Grill Dehydrate 90C, Ninja Foodie Bake 110C
2. Grind the mixed nuts, mixed seeds, and chia seeds to a fine powder
3. Put all the dry ingredients into a large bowl and mix
4. Add the water and melted butter to the bowl and mix. It should look like damp sand....almost the texture of sand when you are about to build a sandcastle :-) * If your seed mix is linseed dominated, add a little more water, maybe 10-20g more
5. Let it rest for 5 minutes
6. Press into your desired shapes; I used a falafel maker and made them no more than 1cm thick (if you go thicker, you will need to extend your cooking time
7. Transfer to a lined Baking tray
8. Cook at 120C, for approx 1 hour, maybe a little more. We are drying out the biscuits, not cooking - This is important. When you snap one in half, if it looks moist, cooks for a little longer
9. If you are cooking in the Ninja foodie, cook at 110C for approx.1 hour, or in the Ninja Grill, on Dehydrate at 90C for 2 to 2 1/2 hours

Lemon Cake

Sweet Treat Recipe | **Prep Time:** 15 minutes | **Servings:** 16

Per Serving: Kcal: 101, Carbs (net) 2.6 grams, Protein 2.8 grams, Fat 9.2 grams

Ingredients
- 110g Unsalted Butter, softened
- 30g Truvia / Natvia / Pure Via Sweetener
- 3 Large Eggs (increase to 4 eggs if making the nut free cake)
- 25g Coconut Flour (increase to 40g if making the nut free cake)
- 50g Ground Almonds (omit these and add the extra egg & coconut flour for nut free cake)
- 1 tsp Baking Powder
- 70g Greek or Greek-Style Yogurt
- 1 tsp Vanilla Extract
- Juice & Zest of 2 wax-free lemons

Directions
1. Preheat the oven to 190°C.
2. Cream the softened butter and sweetener together.
3. Add one egg at a time to the butter and mix thoroughly before adding the next one.
4. Add the coconut flour, ground almonds, and baking powder. Combine with the butter/egg mix.
5. Add the yogurt, vanilla, lemon juice & lemon zest and mix again. DON'T WORRY - the mix will look weird (like a scrambled egg!). This is normal. See the video at the bottom of this page to see if your cake mix looks like ours.
6. Pour the mix into either a lined 8" square tin or divide into 16 silicone muffin cases. Bake for 20-25 minutes (this could be less if making the muffins). Once baked, let the cake cool completely before removing it from the tray/cases.
7. To make a lemon drizzle to top the cake, mix 1 tbsp Greek or Greek-Style Yogurt, 1 tsp Truvia / Natvia / Pure Via Sweetener, and 1 tsp lemon juice. Spread thinly across the top of the cake.

Lemon Curd

Sweet Treat Recipe | **Prep Time:** 15 minutes | **Servings:** 25
Per Serving: Kcal: 55, Carbs (net) 2.3 grams, Protein 0.9 grams, Fat 4.9 grams

Ingredients
- 120ml Lemon Juice
- 2 tbsp Lemon Zest
- 100g Xylitol, ground to a powder
- 120g Melted Unsalted Butter
- 2 Medium Eggs
- 3 Medium Egg Yolks

- 1/2 tsp Salt

Directions
1. Whisk the eggs and egg yolks together using an electric whisk
2. Add the sweetener and whisk for 2 minutes
3. Add all remaining ingredients and mix
4. Microwave this for 1 minute.
5. Use a spatula to beat the mixture.
6. Repeat steps 4 and 5 three more times - the mixture will thicken on the last one
7. Store the lemon curd in the fridge for 7-10 days or freeze

Marzipan Biscuits

Sweet Treat Recipe | **Prep Time:** 15 minutes | **Servings:** 15
Per Serving: Kcal: 103, Carbs (net) 1 gram, Protein 4.2 grams, Fat 8.8 grams

Ingredients
- 300g Ground Almonds (or other ground nuts/seeds - ground pecans work nicely). To mill these, simply blitz them in a Nutri-bullet style blender for just a few seconds.
- 60g Truvia / Natvia / Pure Via Sweetener
- 2 Medium Egg Yolks
- 40-60ml Water
- Flavoring of choice: 1 tsp Almond Essence or Vanilla Extract, or add a spice, e.g. 1 tsp Mixed Spice or 1 tsp, Ground Ginger

Directions
1. Preheat the oven to 200°C.
2. Add all ingredients to a bowl and beat them until the dough ball forms.
3. Roll out the dough between greaseproof / silicone sheets.
4. Use a cookie cutter to cut out your biscuits and place them on an oven tray lined with greaseproof baking paper. To make hanging decorations like the ones in a photo, make a hole in the dough with a straw.
5. Bake for around 15 minutes until slightly crispy. They will be crispy more as they cool. Keep an eye on them to make sure they don't burn!

Microwave Cookie

Sweet Treat Recipe | **Prep Time:** 5 minutes | **Servings:** 2
Per Serving: Kcal: 313, Fat 28 grams, Protein 9.4 grams, Carbs (net) 4.3 grams

Ingredients

- 15g Coconut Oil
- 1 Egg Yolk
- 1/2 tsp Vanilla Essence
- 55g Ground Almonds
- 25g Truvia / Natvia / Pure Via Sweetener
- 10g Choc Chips (we use chopped up 85% dark chocolate)

Directions
1. Melt the coconut oil and allow it to cool for a moment.
2. Add all the other ingredients to this and mix well until a crumble texture forms.
3. Now use your hands to form a dough ball.
4. Grease a microwave plate or line with greaseproof paper.
5. Cut the dough ball in half.
6. Take one half of the dough ball and press it onto a plate to create a cookie shape.
7. Cook one cookie in the microwave for 30 seconds. Cook for a further 30 seconds.
8. Allow to cool and repeat with the second cookie.

Millionaire's Brownie Cake

Sweet Treat Recipe | **Prep Time:** 15 minutes | **Servings:** 12
Per Serving: Kcal: 301, 4.5g Carbs, 5.2g Protein, 28.4g Fat

Ingredients
- 1 batch of Chocolate Brownies
- 2 batches of Butterscotch Sauce
- 100g 85% Dark Chocolate
- 20g Butter

Optional Extras
- Chocolate bits
- Chopped nuts

Directions
1. Make up the Chocolate Brownies recipe according to the recipe instructions & add any of the optional extras (:-))
2. Once the cake is out of the oven - leave it in the tin
3. Make up the Butterscotch Sauce according to the recipe instructions. If you want the sauce a little thicker, add a couple of extra Sugar-Free Werthers (the hard-boiled ones) - This sauce will thicken as it cools
4. Pour all the butterscotch sauce with the cake into the tin and completely cover the brownie cake's top. Allow to cool slightly, before the final step

5. Break up all the chocolate into a microwave bowl and add the butter. Melt in 30-sec blasts until almost melted. Then stir till melted and smooth. Allow cooling for a couple of minutes
6. Pour completely, covering the butterscotch sauce.
7. Once the chocolate is set, it's ready!
8. Enjoy :-)

No-Bake Cheesecake

Sweet Treat Recipe | **Prep Time:** 15 minutes | **Servings:** 12
Per Serving: Kcal: 315, Carbs (net) 2.4 grams, Protein 5.4 grams, Fat 31.5 grams

Ingredients
- 100g Unsalted Butter
- 190g Ground Almonds (or other milled nuts/seeds)
- 30g Truvia / Natvia / Pure Via Sweetener
- 1 Sachet Hartley's Sugar-free Jelly Powder
- 120ml Boiling Water
- 200g Soft Cream Cheese
- 300ml Double Cream
- 80g Frozen Strawberries / Raspberries (defrosted)

Directions
1. Melt the butter in a pan or large bowl in the microwave.
2. Add the sweetener and ground almonds and mix until all the almonds are combined.
3. Line an 8" springform cake tin with grease-proof paper and press the base into the tin. Place in the fridge or freezer while you make the topping.
4. Mix the jelly sachet with 120ml boiling water and stir to dissolve the jelly fully.
5. Using either a hand whisk or a food mixer, combine the cream cheese and double cream until thick, and then slowly add the jelly mix.
6. Add the berries and then mix again for a few seconds.
7. Spoon the topping onto the base and smooth with the back of a spoon or spatula.
8. Allow setting in the fridge for at least an hour.

Rhubarb & Ginger Cake

Sweet Treat Recipe | **Prep Time:** 15 minutes | **Servings:** 8
Per Serving: Kcal: 221, Carbs (net) 2 grams, Protein 8 grams, Fat 20 grams

Ingredients
- 3 Large Eggs
- 70g Unsalted Butter, melted & cooled
- 1 tsp Ground Ginger
- 1 tsp Baking Powder
- 1/2 tsp Vanilla Extract
- 25g Truvia / Natvia / Pure Via Sweetener
- 150g Ground Almonds
- 150g Fresh Rhubarb, trimmed and cut into 2-3cm chunks

Directions
1. Preheat the oven to 180°C.
2. In a large bowl, whisk the eggs and slowly add the melted butter - use an electric whisk if possible, as this will help make the cake light and fluffy.
3. Continue to whisk and add the ginger, baking powder, vanilla extract, and sweetener.
4. Finally, add the ground almonds and whisk.
5. Add half of the rhubarb chunks to the mix and pour it into a lined 6-7" cake tin.
6. Add the remaining rhubarb to the top of the cake.
7. Bake for 25-30 minutes. If you have a Ninja Foodi, bake directly on the base at 175°C for 20 minutes.

Rosie's Mug Cake

Sweet Treat Recipe | **Prep Time:** 5 minutes | **Servings:** 1
Per Serving: Kcal: 455, 5.9g Carbs, 16g Protein, 40.3g Fat

Ingredients
- 15g Unsalted Butter
- 30g Soft Cream Cheese
- 30g Ground Almonds
- 5g Truvia / Natvia / Pure Via Sweetener
- 1 Large Egg
- 1/2 tsp Vanilla Extract
- 1/2 tsp Baking Powder

Directions
1. Add the butter to a microwaveable mug small dish and microwave for around 15 seconds at a time until melted.
2. Add the remaining ingredients (adjust the sweetener to taste) and mix.
3. Microwave on full power for one minute, allow it to settle slightly, and then microwave for another minute.

Spiced Easter Buns

Sweet Treat Recipe | **Prep Time:** 20 minutes | **Servings:** 10

Per Serving: Kcal: 159, 3.9g Carbs, 7.5g Protein, 11.8g Fat

Ingredients

- 180g Milled Golden Linseed
- 100g Ground Almonds
- 3 tsp Baking Powder
- 1 sachet (7g) Fast Acting Dried Yeast
- 25g Truvia / Natvia / Pure Via Sweetener (adjust to taste)
- 2-3 tbsp Mixed Spice (adjust to taste)
- 6 Large Eggs
- 180ml Warm Water
- 1 tsp Vanilla Extract
- Optional: 25g Dried Currants (we chop these up into smaller pieces)
- Optional: 50g 85% Dark Chocolate, finely chopped

Directions

1. Preheat the oven to 180°C.
2. Mix the linseed, almonds, yeast, baking powder, sweetener, and spice in a large bowl. Add the currants if you're using them.
3. Add the eggs, vanilla, and water. Mix until smooth.
4. Check the temperature of the mix before adding the chocolate (you don't want it to melt while you're mixing).
5. Set the mix aside for 10-15 minutes, allowing it to thicken.
6. The mix should now be quite gloopy - take a spoon of mix and place it on an oven tray lined with greaseproof paper. The mix should hold its shape. Alternatively, divide the mix into small individual tins or silicone muffin cases. Or, pour the whole mix into a lined loaf tin (we use an 8" long tin). We grated some dark chocolate over the top of our loaf before baking :D
7. Bake the individual rolls for around 20 minutes or the loaf for 40-50 minutes, until firm to touch. To give it a nice crust, you may want to take the bread out of its tins/cases for the last 5-10 minutes of baking.
8. Allow the bread to cool slightly before slicing and spreading lots of butter on :D

Mixed Spice Cake

Sweet Treat Recipe | **Prep Time:** 15 minutes | **Servings:** 12
Per Serving: Kcal: 142, 5g Carbs, 5.9g Protein, 10.5g Fat

Ingredients

- 210g Almond Butter (100% nuts)
- 2 Large Eggs
- 40g Dates, blitzed in a little hot water to create a paste.
- 10g Chia Seeds
- 7g Bicarbonate of Soda
- 3 tsp Mixed Spice
- 15g Truvia / Natvia / Pure Via Sweetener
- 25ml/g Lemon Juice

Directions

1. Preheat the oven to 180°C.
2. In a large mixing bowl, combine the almond butter and eggs to create a paste.
3. Add the date puree, chia seeds, bicarbonate of soda, mixed spice, and sweetener.
4. Combine well, and then add the lemon juice. The mix will start to create foam as the lemon juice reacts with the bicarbonate of soda. Keep mixing until all the foam is fully combined.
5. Line a 7" round cake tin and pour the mix in.
6. Bake for 20-25 minutes until firm. This may sink slightly in the middle.

CONCLUSION

One of the main keys to any successful diet or lifestyle change has always been the recipes that fit in with the principles of the diet. There are many ways to achieve ketosis and attain that weight loss goal. However, you do not want to get there by repeatedly having the same old dishes.

Variety is the name of the game here, which is crucial in ensuring the sustainability of the ketogenic diet. With the flavorful and delicious recipes found in this step-by-step keto cookbook, they will be useful additions for any keto dieter at any stage of their ketogenic journey. I have yet to see anyone complain about having too many easy yet delicious recipes!

It would be useful for beginners who have gotten this recipe cookbook to take the 28-day meal plan as a helpful guide. Still, you should step out from that comfort zone sooner or later as you progress along your keto adventure! This is what the multiple recipes are for to pick and choose the most attractive to your palate.

ONE LAST THING...

If you enjoyed this book or found it useful, I'd be very grateful if you'd post a short review on Amazon. Your support makes a difference, and I read all the reviews personally to get your feedback and improve this book.

Thanks again for your support!

Printed in Great Britain
by Amazon